My Healthier Happy Diabetes Journey

My Healthier Happy Diabetes Journey

Shira Niru

Introduction

This e-book is about my struggles, research, experience, and, eventually, my day-to-day success with managing my diabetes. I was diagnosed in 1999 with blood sugar levels of over three hundred, and my doctor prescribed medication. However, it took me several years after that to take and view diabetes seriously. I was fifty-two, and neuropathy, vision, and kidney problems had begun. Starting that year, I made it my life's goal to conquer my diabetes. I sought help from my older aunts and uncles and other elderly folk, but mostly from my grandmother, who knew powerful natural remedies that would keep diabetes under control. When I was a child, my grandmother would give me and my siblings what we called at the time "bush medicine" for all types of ailments, so I knew she was the perfect source to turn to for my research. In doing so, I was able to experiment and experience the effects of herbal products on my diabetes for years.

The information on herbs and spices added to my foods, drinking the teas until I settled on a few favorites, and using diabetes-friendly oils to prepare my dishes helped me conquer my diabetes one day at a time. I have used this method for almost 11 years. There are three more e-books to follow.

Living with diabetes is a struggle that can be daunting and overwhelming. The constant monitoring of blood sugar levels, strict dietary restrictions, and remembering to take medications and exercise in a fast-paced life can seem like a never-ending battle. However, what if I told you that adding some herbs and spices to your life could help control diabetes? Yes, you read that right!

Many cultures have used herbal products for their medicinal properties for generations, and modern research has shown their effectiveness in managing diabetes. Let us explore the excellent benefits they hide and how you can incorporate them into your daily meals to help you control and manage diabetes.

A diabetes diagnosis means that your body's pancreas, or the endocrine pancreas, is not producing sufficient insulin, or whatever it produces is ineffective. The hormone insulin significantly affects how glucose is absorbed and regulated into the bloodstream. When insulin's role is effective, it allows glucose to be transported to cells for energy; however, when it is insufficient, then blood sugar will remain in the blood, and this causes blood sugar levels to become extremely high, which leads to a diagnosis of diabetes and eventual diabetes complications.

The impacts of diabetes are far-reaching and can cause other major health problems. A common diabetic complication is neuropathy, or damaged nerves that often present pain, tingling, and numbness in the hands and feet and can significantly impact a person's quality of life, not to mention the possibility of later limb amputations.

Another significant complication of diabetes is kidney disease. The kidneys' role is to remove excessive fluids and get rid of waste from the body. However, untreated, and uncontrolled high blood sugar levels can cause damage to the kidney's tiny blood vessels, which leads to improper kidney function and kidney failure. Controlling blood sugar and HbA1c levels is vital to manage diabetes and prevent complications.

Moreover, another complication is diabetic retinopathy. This can happen when your blood pressure and cholesterol are high, along with having diabetes. It means that you can develop unhealthy eyes and

vision problems that could result in blindness. Besides being in a physician's care, diabetic retinopathy can be prevented by thoroughly managing diabetes.

Additionally, diabetes can increase the risk of cardiovascular diseases, which can lead to heart attacks and stroke. Everyone with diabetes is at risk because this can deteriorate blood vessels, which leads to poor blood circulation and increases the development of heart disease. People with diabetes are also prone to high blood pressure and abnormal cholesterol levels, further aggravating the risk of cardiovascular problems.

Furthermore, diabetes will have a dangerous and negative impact on mental health. The diagnosis of diabetes, along with the potential complications, can contribute to overall stress, anxiety, and depression. Individuals with diabetes need to prioritize managing diabetes and their mental well-being. Ask your doctor for help and talk with your family and friends for support.

Educate yourself and understand the impacts and complications of diabetes. It is pivotal in managing this chronic illness effectively. By controlling and managing blood sugar levels, you can minimize and even prevent the risk of neuropathy, kidney disease, eye and vision disease, cardiovascular problems, gum disease, and other related complications.

Besides the health advantages mentioned about each herbal product, some or all have more benefits. Still, this e-book focuses on controlling and managing diabetes and preventing or reducing the risks of this chronic disease. While herbs, spices, teas, and oils can provide benefits in managing diabetes, they cannot cure the condition. Diabetes (the killer beast) is life-threatening and requires ongoing management and medical supervision.

However, incorporating certain herbs, spices, teas, and oils into your meal routine can help control blood sugar and minimize complications. In this e-book, let us dig deeper into these natural remedies' nutritional value and healing power and how they can positively impact diabetes management. And add exercise to your daily routine.

Gain control of your blood sugar levels in a way only **YOU** can. Read on to discover how to unlock the potential of herbal products used in Ayurvedic medicine on your journey to control diabetes naturally!

A word of warning: Please consult your healthcare provider before trying the products mentioned in this e-book, especially if you have never eaten or drank them before.

Tips to Help You Get Started

Educate Yourself: Get to know the nutritional value of different herbs, spices, teas, and oils for diabetes control. Learning about the components of herbal products, what they are, how they work, and how they benefit diabetes can help you make informed choices and create your personalized plan.

Speak With Your Healthcare Provider: Before integrating herbal products into your daily cooking, consult with your healthcare professional. Ask questions about safety and interaction with other medications you are currently taking. They can help you create a care plan suited just for you.

Start Slow: To introduce herbs, spices, into your diet, begin using small amounts and increase the amount gradually over time. Monitor your sugar levels before and after to note any reactions and side effects.

Try different recipes: Incorporating herbs and spices into your everyday meals can be fun and interesting. Try cooking different foods using herbs and spices, and what works best for you.

Monitor Your Blood Sugar Levels: Check your blood sugar before eating foods incorporated with herbal products and after eating. Keep a daily log of which herbal products are best for you.

Be Consistent: Do not start today and skip tomorrow, you must be consistent if you want to see results. Incorporate them into your daily cooking routine and a regular addition of your meals. This must become a lifestyle for long-term benefits.

Also, each person's experience with herbal products may not be the same. Experiment, find out what works best for you. Also, if you are a smoker, quit. Alcohol and diabetes are a dangerous combination. Quit drinking alcohol if you do. Avoid sweetened beverages and food. Get in the right mindset to adjust to living a life with diabetes. Use these guidelines to help you on your journey to manage diabetes naturally with the power of herbs, spices, teas, and oils. Try new things, be bold, and most importantly, enjoy the herbal journey towards better health!

Herbal Products to Treat Diabetes

Food high in antioxidants and anti-inflammatory properties are powerful in fighting diabetes and its complications. All the herbs, spices, teas, and oils mentioned in this e-book have components, compounds, or properties that, in one way or another, can and may tremendously assist the person with diabetes in controlling blood sugar levels and improving Hemoglobin A1c levels. Dealing with diabetes is challenging, but consistently incorporating these herbal products into your daily meal routine could provide significant benefits in controlling blood sugar levels and preventing diabetes complications. For example, turmeric contains curcumin, which reduces inflammation and oxidative stress, protecting nerves from damage and reducing the risk of neuropathy. Additionally, cinnamon can improve peripheral neuropathy by encouraging insulin sensitivity and regulating blood sugar levels.

Another crucial aspect to consider is kidney health. Certain herbal products have beneficial effects on kidney health. For instance, dandelion root tea (containing antioxidants) has diuretic properties that promote urine production, helping flush out kidney toxins. Furthermore, ginger (which contains antioxidants) helps to reduce kidney inflammation and protect against kidney disease caused by diabetes. The healing power of herbal commodities in controlling diabetes extends beyond neuropathy and kidney health. These natural remedies have promoted insulin sensitivity, lowered blood sugar levels, and reduced inflammation.

Some examples include fenugreek, bitter melon (a superfood), and garlic. Fenugreek seeds help to lower blood glucose levels and improve glucose tolerance when consumed raw, roasted, or added to meals. Garlic has properties that may reduce inflammation and promote insulin sensitivity, making it an excellent spice for diabetes management.

Bitter melon, a diabetic superfood, is a vegetable commonly used in traditional medicine. It contains compounds that mimic insulin's effects, helping regulate blood sugar levels. From reducing neuropathy symptoms to protecting kidney and heart health, these natural remedies offer a holistic approach to diabetes management. Let's take a deeper look into the benefits and nutritional value of herbs, spices, teas, and oils for you.

Table of Contents

Introduction III

Tips to Help You Get Started I

Herbal Products to Treat Diabetes II

Marjoram Benefits & Uses.. 1

Marjoram Tea & Oil.. 2

Benefits of Sage 3

Sage Oil & Tea... 4

Benefits & Uses of Basil 5

Basil Tea & Oil 6

Rosemary's Uses & Benefits 7

Rosemary Tea & Oil.. 8

Oregano's Uses & Benefits 9

Oregano Tea & Oil... 10

Thyme Benefits 11

Thyme Tea & Oil.. 12

Dill's Health Benefits 13

Parsley & Its Roots 14

Tarragon's Health Benefits.. 15

Bay Leaves Benefits & Uses 16

Lemon Balm 17

Benefits of Fenugreek.. 18

Benefits of Leek 19

Fennel's Benefits.. 20

Green Onion's/Scallions 21

Cilantro Benefits.. 22

How About Culantro?... 23

Diabetic Benefits of Onions 24

Chives 25

Savory's Benefits 26

A History Bit of & Herbs & Spices 27

A Little of My History 28

Garlic's Diabetic Benefits 29

Ginger's Benefits 30

Turmeric's Diabetic Benefits...31

Health Benefits of Flaxseeds 32

Health Benefits of Cinnamon 33

Nutmeg's Benefits 34

Benefits In Cloves..35

Paprika's Diabetic Benefits 36

Health Benefits in Cumin 37

Cardamon Spice 38

Chamomile Tea & Oil...39

Dandelion's Benefits 40

Mauby Bark Drink Benefits 41

Black Tea's Benefits...42

Green Tea Benefits...43

Rooibos Tea Benefits..44

Oolong Tea Benefits...45

Benefits in Mint Tea 46

Ginseng Tea..47

Mulberry Leaf Tea 48

Moringa Leaf Tea 49

Aloe Vera Benefits..50

Mango Leaf Benefits 52

Guava Leaf Benefits 53

Bitterwood Leaf Tea...54

Java Plum Leaf Tea..55

Shatter Stone Leaf Tea...56

Neem Tea Benefits..57

African Bitter Leaf Tea...58

Pine Bark/Needles Tea...59

Banaba Tea Benefits... 60

Gymnema Sylvestre Benefits 61

European Bilberry Tea..62

Sorrel/Hibiscus/ Roselle Drink 63

Loquat/Japanese Plum Tea Benefits.......................................64

Benefits of Milk Thistle 65

Berberine Tea...66

Bitter Melon/Gourd Leaf Tea 67

Benefits of Stevia... 68

Monk Fruit as a Sugar Substitute...69

Avocado & Extra Virgin Olive Oil 70

Sesame & Rice Bran Oil... 71

Almond & Walnut Oil 72

Grapeseed & Macadamia Oil...73

Safflower & Peanut Oil..74

Hazelnut & Pecan Oil 75

Chestnut & Coconut Virgin Oil 76

Pistachio Nut Oil, Brazil Nut Oil, Cashew Nut Oil 77

Peppers For Diabetes 78

Author's Notes 79

Disclaimer 80

Author's Letter 81

Author's Profile..82

Marjoram Benefits & Uses

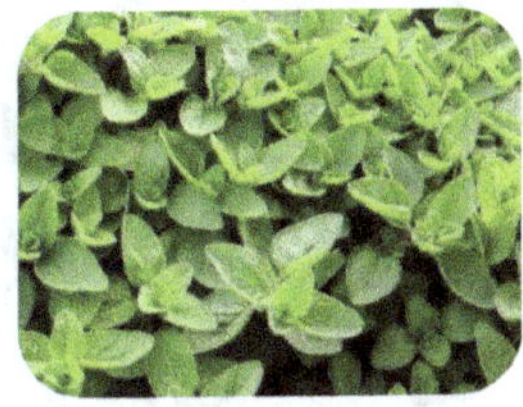

Fresh Marjoram (Design by Pixabay)

Marjoram is rich in compounds and has been used as traditional and home medicine. Certain cultures believe that marjoram is a natural and safe treatment for diabetes. In addition to antioxidants, anti-inflammatory, and anti-microbial compounds, it contains minerals, vitamins, enzymes, and other nutrients, which offer a variety of health benefits.

Carvacrol, an antioxidant found in marjoram stimulates insulin sensitivity and helps regulate normal blood sugar levels. It also has significant health properties that boost the immune system, improve mental health, protect the cardiovascular and circulatory systems, and reduce the risks of chronic diseases. Its natural diuretic properties mean that it can help lower high blood pressure, and its antibacterial properties can aid in the healing of gastrointestinal ulcers.

Use 1/2 to 1 teaspoon of fresh, dried, or crushed marjoram leaves to flavor the food. It is excellent in soups, stews, salads, sauces, meats, curries, vegetables, fish, and seafood. Sprinkle it on side dishes. Use moderately. Add it to food towards the end of cooking to retain its flavor, or you can wrap one to two teaspoons of marjoram in a small cheesecloth and add it to the pot while cooking stews, soups, and sauces.

Marjoram Tea & Oil

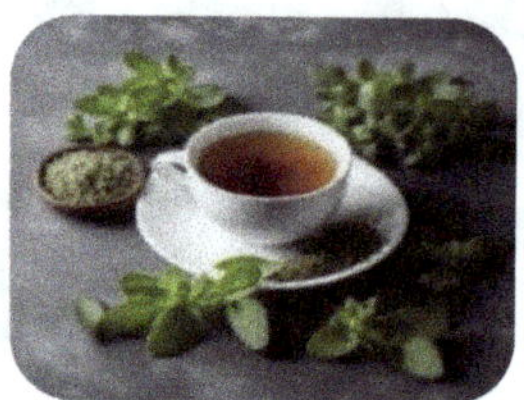

Marjoram Tea (Designed by Freepik)

For a tasty and flavorful cup of marjoram tea, use 2.5 cups pure filtered water, 1 tbsp dried marjoram, 1/4 tsp fresh ginger, 1/2 tsp cinnamon, 1-2 stevia leaves or recommended amount of pure extract (your choice). Stevia is extremely sweet so use less. Boil the water, add cinnamon, boil for 2 minutes; add other ingredients and cook for another minute. Allow the brew to steep for 8-10 minutes, strain, and drink.

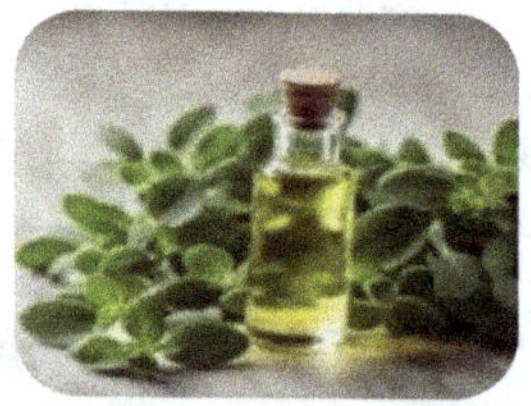

Marjoram Oil (Designed by Freepik)

Marjoram oil helps with relaxation, mood, and sleep. Drizzle it over salads. Mix it with rosemary, lavender, cypress, or other therapeutic oils in a diffuser to experience its beautiful aromas, calming effects, and other benefits. It is very soothing when rubbed on any part of the body. My grandmother grew this herb in her greenhouse garden and brewed it for its calming and restful sleep effects.

Benefits of Sage

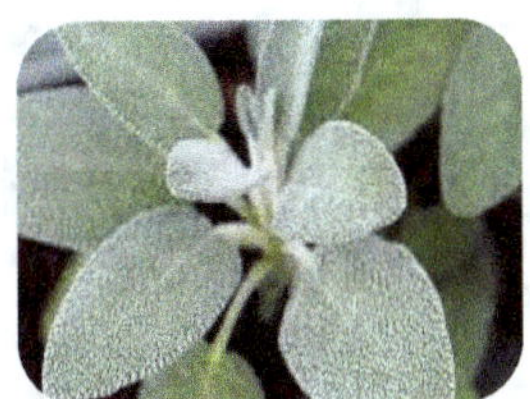

Sage Leaves (Design by Pixabay)

Many cultures have used sage leaves to treat diabetes symptoms and for culinary purposes for centuries. Sage leaves are packed with vitamins, nutrients, anti-cancer, anti-inflammatory, anti-bacterial, and several antioxidant compounds that contribute to impressive health benefits. Certain antioxidants in sage may lower blood sugar levels, clear fatty acids in the blood, encourage insulin sensitivity and production and transport blood sugar into cells (and not into the bloodstream) for energy, thereby regulating glucose levels.

Additional health advantages include the reduction of bad cholesterol, better blood circulation, and improved heart health. Moreover, consuming sage extract may protect against brain diseases like Alzheimer's and improve brain functions. In addition, it might lower the chance of developing some cancers, including those of the liver, kidney, breast, colon, and cervix.

Sage should only be used sparingly in cuisines because of its potent flavor and potential to reduce blood sugar. It is available in whole, ground, or dried leaf form. Use 1/2 teaspoon finely chopped sage sprinkled on roast dishes and meats, squash, vegetables, soups, stews, and sauces.

Sage Oil & Tea

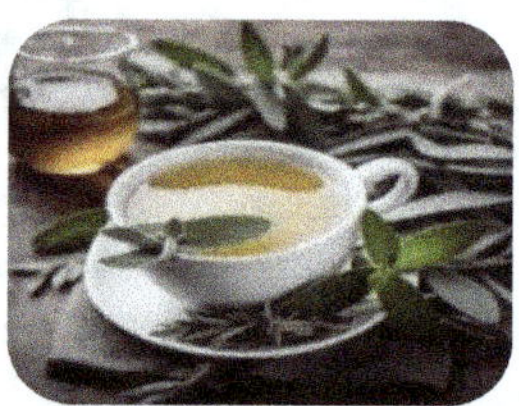

Sage Tea (Designed by Freepik)

Sage tea may improve blood sugar and HbA1c levels and prevent after-meal spikes. To make sage tea, use one teaspoon of dried sage or one tablespoon of freshly chopped sage, one cup of pure filtered water, add sage, and boil for 1 minute; use a sweetener like stevia; I usually add one stevia leaf and a mint leaf, which is also diabetic-friendly to the boiling water with the sage. It enhances the flavor of the tea for me. Let steep for 4-5 minutes, strain, add a slice of lemon, and enjoy.

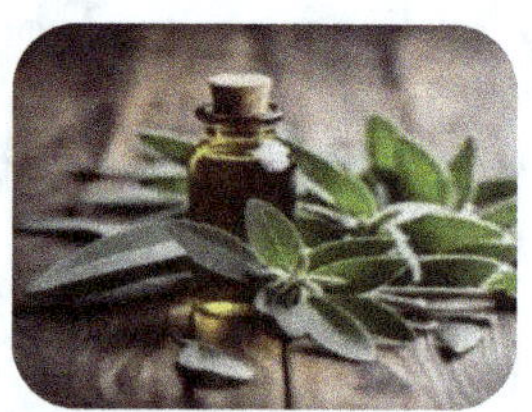

Sage Oil (Designed by Freepik)

Do not apply sage oil or any essential oil directly to the skin. Add carrier oil, mix well, and then apply to the skin for a massage. To clean the air of bacteria in your home or office and enjoy calming effects, add three drops of sage oil, eight ounces of water, and one ounce of other essential oils in an oil diffuser.

Benefits & Uses of Basil

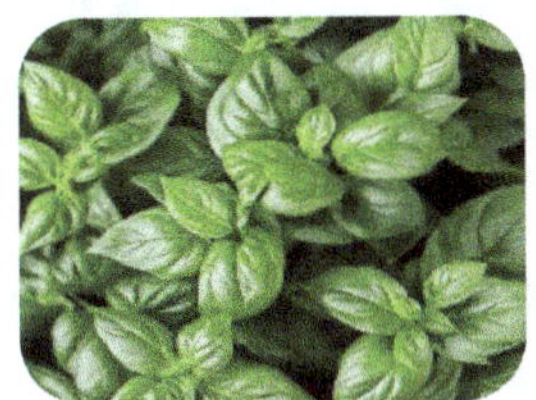

Fresh Basil (Designed by Freepik)

There are several types of basil, such as garden basil, holy basil, sweet basil, and purple basil, to name a few. Basil is a popular herb used in cuisines around the world. It is rich in vitamins, minerals, nutrients, anti-hyperglycemic activities, and anti-inflammatory, anti-cancer, and antioxidants that host impressive health benefits.

Basil contains phenolic compounds that contribute to anti-hyperglycemic activities that may help lower high blood sugar levels and prevent the long-term effects of diabetes. Regular consumption may protect against cell damage and prevent chronic illnesses, including cancer. Basil's plant compounds may help regulate blood pressure, lower cholesterol, and triglyceride levels. In addition, other health benefits could include heart and cardiovascular health, improved blood circulation, and a stronger immune system.

Basil makes a flavorful addition to many different dishes. Fresh basil is the best to use in food because you will get the full benefits. Use finely chopped basil in stews, soups, sauces, curries, fish, seafood, vegetables, salads, and side dishes. Mince or chop it with other herbs to rub on all meats, even turkey; add it to stuffed dishes. However, use basil in moderation.

Basil Tea & Oil

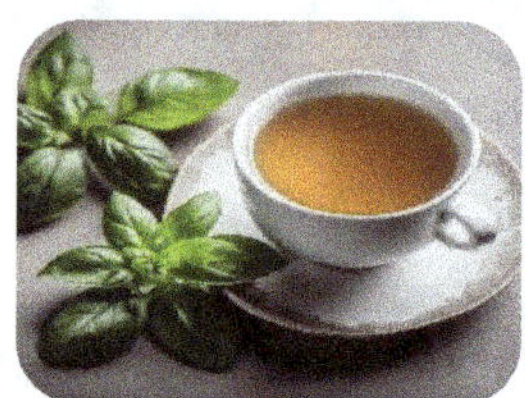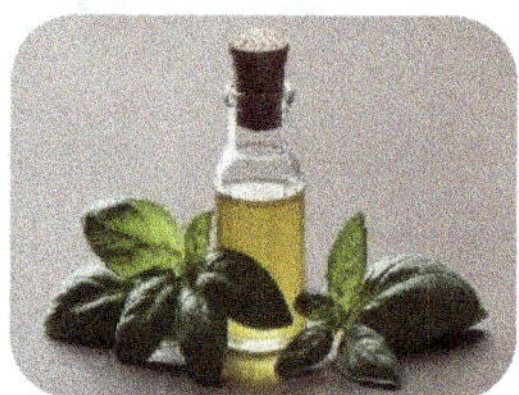

Basil Tea & Oil (Designed by Freepik)

Basil tea is rare, but it is brewed and consumed in various parts of the world because of its dense nutrients, antioxidant content, and impressive health benefits. It also helps keep diabetic symptoms under control and aids in stabilizing blood glucose levels, blood pressure, and lipid profile. It also helps with stress, pain, and oral care.

Boil two cups of filtered water, add 1/2 cup of basil, and boil for 4 minutes. (I usually add a mint leaf, one stevia leaf, and a dash of cinnamon for a better flavor). Strain, drink, and enjoy.

Basil oil has an array of impressive benefits for skin and hair. It treats and cures acne, heals eczema, clears pores of dead cells and other impurities, reduces wrinkles, improves skin complexion, wards off skin irritations, heals wounds and sores, and boosts skin cells metabolism and elasticity. It also removes dandruff, and massaging basil oil with coconut oil on the scalp increases blood flow and promotes healthy hair roots that can help with hair growth. Use basil oil moderately as a dipping oil, and drizzle over salads and vegetables.

Rosemary's Uses & Benefits

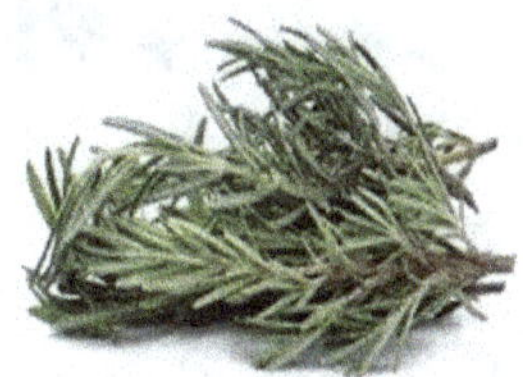

Fresh Rosemary (Designed by Freepik)

Rosemary is rich in impressive antioxidants, anti-inflammatory compounds, anti-cancer, anti-tumor, anti-microbial properties, nutrients, vitamins, and minerals.

The plant's extract and phenolic compound may play a massive role in regulating blood glucose and lipid metabolism. It may also increase insulin sensitivity, which makes it an excellent treatment for diabetes. Additionally, for the diabetic, rosemary's plant health benefits include eye and vision health, proper blood circulation, controlled blood pressure, and a healthy heart and cardiovascular system.

Antioxidants in rosemary help to prevent chronic illnesses such as cancer, heart disease and diabetes. It also boosts immune health and promotes brain health by improving memory and cognitive performance. Rosemary also improves mood and mental alertness. Rosemary is an aromatic herb used in many cuisines all around the world. It adds pleasant flavors to dishes. However, use it in moderation to prevent overpowering other food flavors. Use finely chopped rosemary (2-3 leaves) in stews, sauces, soups, all vegetables, and beans. Add ¼ teaspoon finely chopped rosemary to marinades and seasonings for all meats, fish, and seafood. Mix in casseroles, salads, and stuffed dishes. Use rosemary sparingly.

Rosemary Tea & Oil

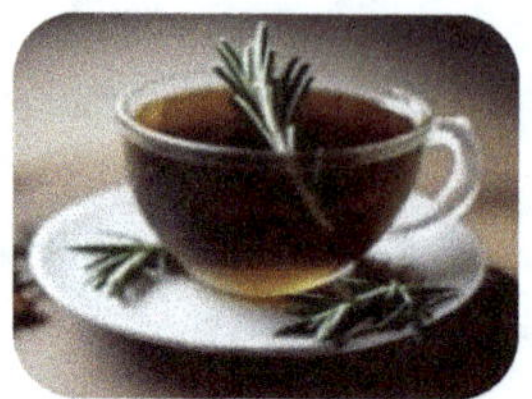

Rosemary Tea (Designed by Picsart)

Besides helping to lower high blood sugar levels, promoting insulin-like production, and absorbing glucose into muscle cells for energy and storage, rosemary tea reduces stress and anxiety, boosts mood, and improves concentration and memory. Unique compounds in basil may prevent neurodegenerative diseases like Alzheimer's and improve overall brain health. It also has eye and vision health benefits. In two cups of filtered boiling water, steep for 4-5 minutes, 1 tbsp dried or 1-2 tsp fresh rosemary, add sweetener (like stevia), strain, and drink.

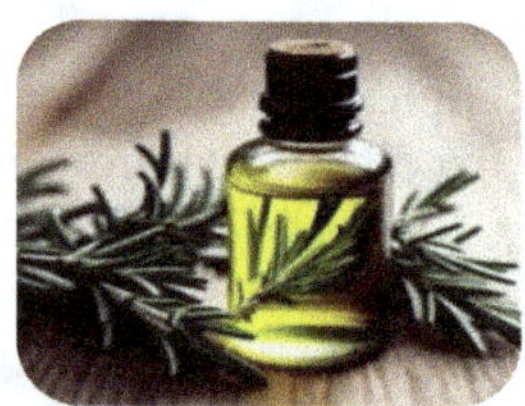

Rosemary Oil (Designed by Picsart)

Breathing rosemary oil may improve focus, concentration, memory, mood, alertness, and energy. It may also improve blood circulation and relieve stress when rubbed on limbs and body. Massaging rosemary oil on the scalp will help with hair loss. It is also a joint pain reliever and bug repellent. Drizzle a small amount on salads.

Oregano's Uses & Benefits

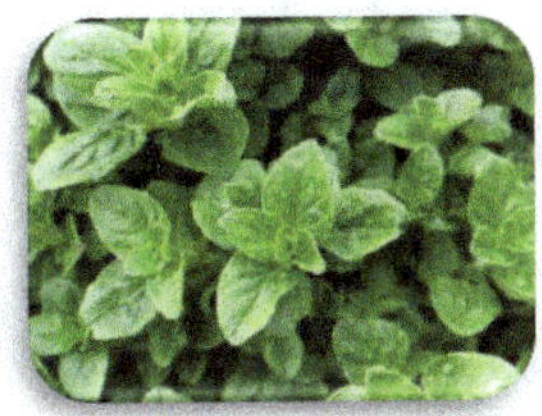

Fresh Oregano (Designed by Pixabay)

Oregano has plant compounds with anti-diabetic properties. Carvacrol helps to regulate blood sugar levels by stimulating insulin production and sensitivity, it may also protect against diabetes, and reduce diabetes complications. In addition, oregano contains antioxidants, anti-inflammatory, and antimicrobial components, vitamins, minerals, and other nutrients that make it valuable in any diet.

Health benefits include protection of the heart and cardiovascular system, lower risk of neuropathy and kidney disease, reduced inflammation in the body, which is helpful for people with diabetes. Furthermore, oregano's extract boosts the immune system and energy levels, improves liver, bone, and digestive health, detoxifies the body, and protects cells from cancer and other damage due to free radicals.

Oregano has a pleasant aroma and flavor, but a strong taste, so it is best to use it sparingly. Add finely chopped oregano to soups, vegetables, sauces, stews, curries, all meat dishes, fish, roasted dishes, and even salads.

Oregano Tea & Oil

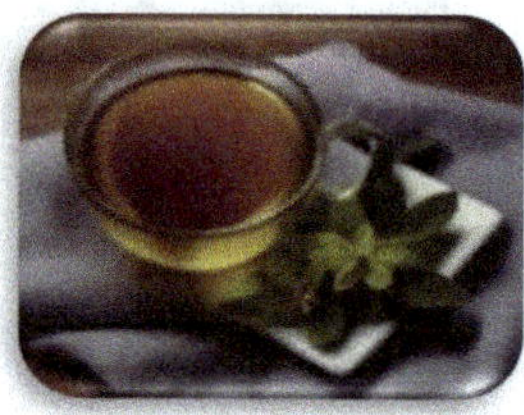

Oregano Tea (Designed by Picsart)

Consuming oregano tea helps promote a healthy heart, cardiovascular system, and bone health and boosts the immune system. It also reduces cancer risk and can help with cough, nausea, digestive problems, sore throat, edema, bloating, and irritable bowel syndrome.

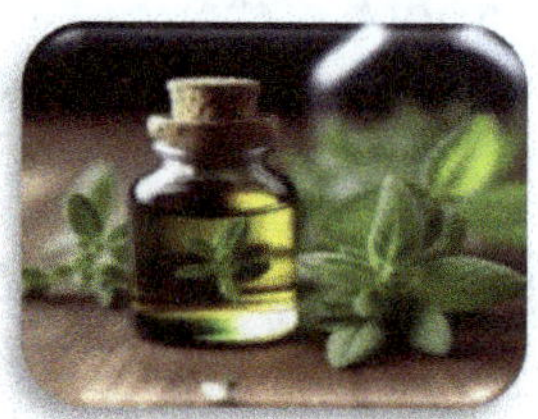

Oregano Oil (Designed by Picsart)

Use oregano oil mixed with coconut or other essential oils to apply to the skin. Some uses include acne, wounds, sores, muscle and joint pain, insect bites, varicose veins, warts, athlete's foot, rosacea, mouth sores, gum disease, psoriasis, and more.

Thyme Benefits

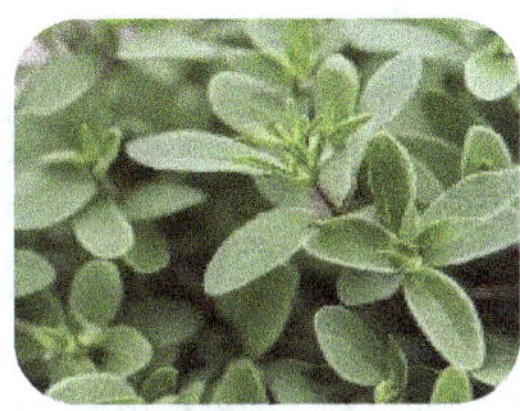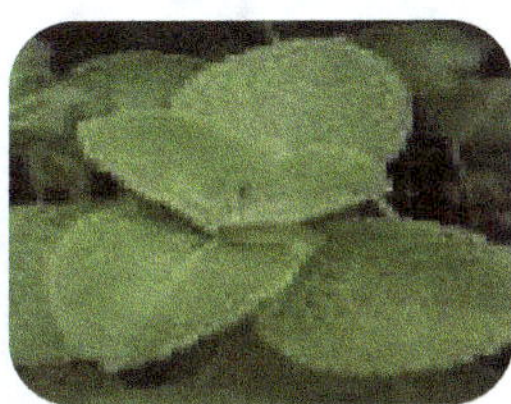

Fine Leaf & Broad Leaf Thyme (Design by Freepik)

Currently there is no known cure for diabetes, but there are ways to control and manage the condition and enjoy overall health. The thyme herb has become popular for its anti-diabetic properties and the potential to help regulate blood sugar levels. Thyme is used by cooks as a seasoning in cuisines worldwide. It contains medicinal properties used to treat various ailments.

Thyme, a versatile herb contains flavonoids, anti-inflammatory, antibacterial, antifungal properties, and other antioxidants that help regulate blood sugar levels, promote insulin sensitivity, and contribute to diabetes management. It is also rich in vitamins and minerals, iron, and manganese.

Additional health benefits include protecting heart, liver, and bone health, lowering blood pressure and cholesterol levels, preventing eye disease, improving blood circulation and cognitive skills, and reducing risk of kidney problems and cancers. There are several varieties of thyme, and each has a distinct aromatic flavor. To reap thyme's benefits incorporate it into your diet. Thyme pairs well with meats, fish, stews, sauces, curries, salads, vegetables, and soups.

Thyme Tea & Oil

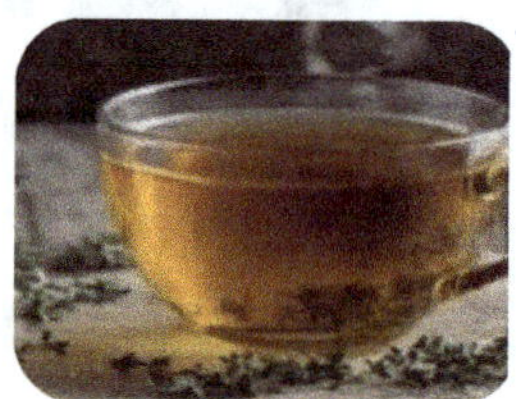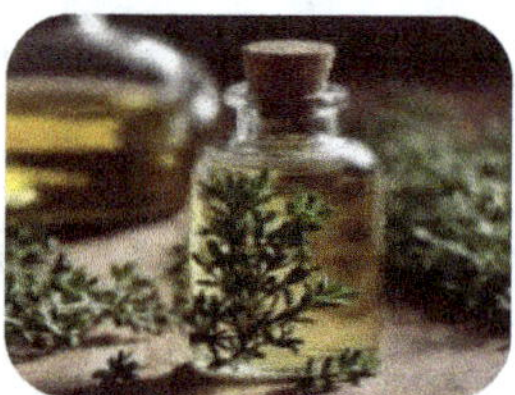

Thyme Tea & Oil (Designed by Freepik)

Thyme tea contains antibacterial, antimicrobial, antifungal, antioxidant properties, essential vitamins, and minerals. Besides many of the benefits mentioned earlier, it may also help with respiratory problems, coughs, and the nervous system. Thyme oil may help with acne, hair loss, breast cancer prevention, and diabetes management. Other benefits may include heart, liver, and bone health.

Do not use undiluted essential oil on your scalp or any skin area; mix with coconut, jojoba, primrose, or grapeseed oil for scalp and skin use. Drizzle thyme oil over salads.

Both fine leaf and broad leaf thyme were a must in seasonings of meats, fish, and seafood at my grandmother's home. Fish and seafood were abundant there because she lived close to Clifton Hill and Sunset Beach. As youngsters, my siblings and I would take nets and catch fish, and when the tide was out, we would take buckets and go out and get conch, clams, chip-chip (small clams), oysters, and there were certain times we caught several varieties of shrimp and crab in abundance. I miss those days.

Dill's Health Benefits

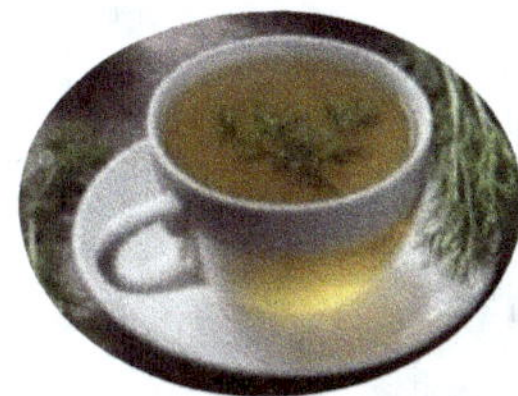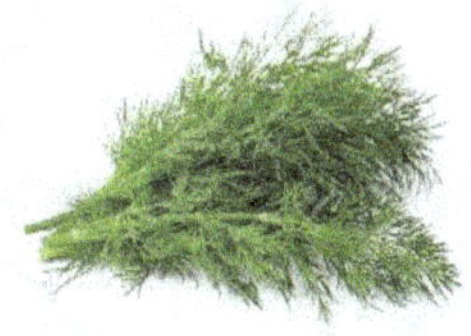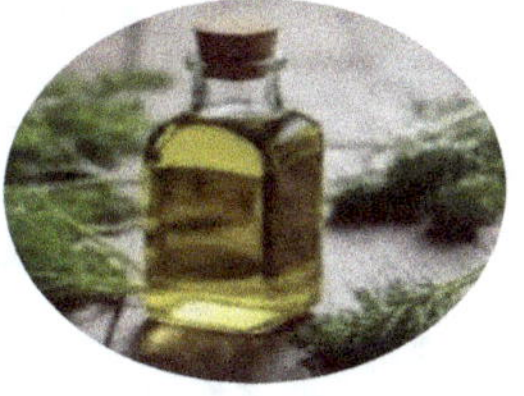

Fresh Dill Tea, Dill, & Oil (Designed by Picsart)

Including dill in your diet can regulate blood sugar levels, balance sugar and fat metabolism in the bloodstream, and support insulin levels. Dill packs a host of antioxidants, vitamins, minerals, and nutrients. Dill weed offers plenty of calcium, iron, and manganese. It is rich in anti-viral, anti-microbial, anti-aging, and anti-inflammatory properties.

Consuming dill improves eye and vision health, boosts the immune system, reduces cholesterol, and helps with respiratory disorders and bone health. It also promotes normal brain functions and improves the nervous system health.

Finely chopped dill adds delicious flavor to many dishes. Use it in stews, casseroles, soups, dips, sauces, ground meat, vegetables, and marinades. Season all meats, fish, and seafood with dill. Add it to salads, vegetables, and fruit smoothies.

Dill tea and oil are known to be suitable for stomach disorders; they aid digestion, prevent infections, help with anxiety and nerves, and help relax muscles.

Parsley & Its Roots

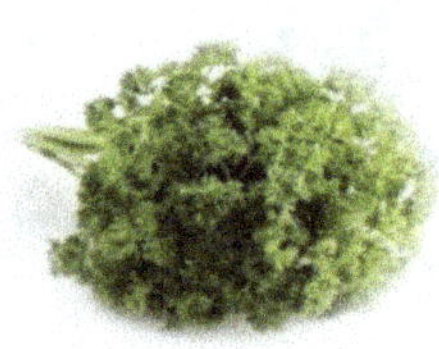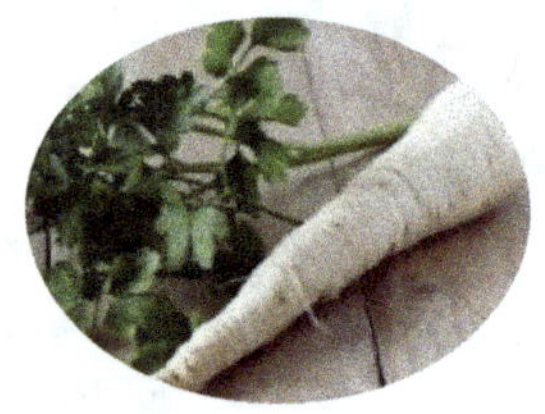

Curly & Flat Leaf Parsley & Parsley Root (Designs by Pixabay)

Another nutritious herb that is high in flavonoids, other antioxidants, vitamins, and minerals, which have several impressive health benefits, is parsley. Certain compounds in parsley could increase insulin production and sensitivity, lower blood sugar levels, and enhance pancreatic functions. Some cultures use parsley as a diabetes medicine.

Additional advantages include kidney and eye health, stomach and uterine health, the prevention of chronic diseases, bone and brain health, and lower cholesterol and blood pressure. It also promotes heart health, prevents the thickening of arterial walls, boosts the immune system, and guards against free radical damage to cells.

It is best to use fresh parsley in foods to extract its full flavor and nutrients. Add chopped parsley with other herbs to season meats, fish, and seafood. Use it in soups, stews, sauces, pasta, dips, salads, sandwiches, curries, vegetables, and smoothies.

Parsley roots flavor dishes with a hint of carrots, celery, and turnip. They can be boiled, steamed, baked, or eaten raw. Add it to stews, soups, salads, and other vegetables for more flavor.

Tarragon's Health Benefits

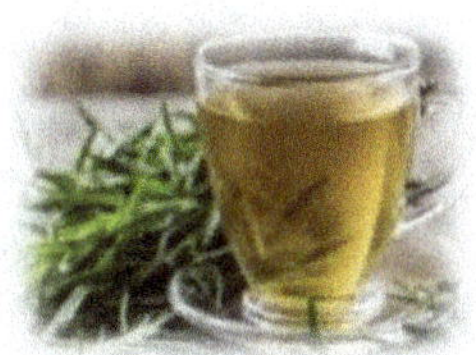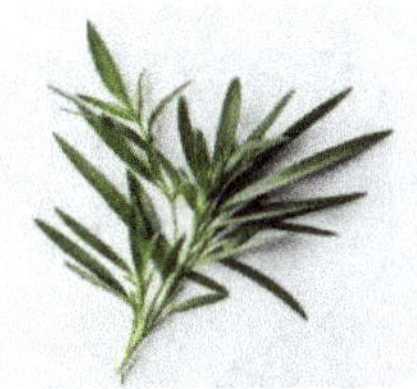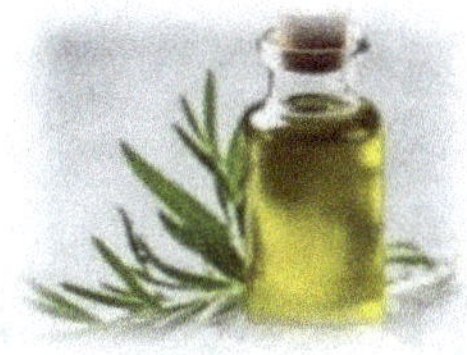

Fresh Tarragon Tea, Leaves & Oil (Design by Pixabay & Freepik)

For a person's blood sugar levels to be normal, all calories, carbohydrates or sugar consumed must be evenly distributed in the body. Tarragon is loaded with compounds and properties that can do just that. The result is improved insulin sensitivity and regulated blood sugar levels.

Other benefits include kidney, heart, liver, vision, brain, and blood circulation health. It also can potentially prevent cancerous cells, fight against bacteria, improve digestive health, and boost the immune system.

Use freshly chopped tarragon in meats, fish, seafood, soups, vegetables, salads, stews, sauces, and eggs.

Tarragon tea and oil also contain the same health benefits as the fresh leaves that are used for seasoning. They also help digestion by breaking down food into essential nutrients, promoting brain functions, and improving the nervous and circulatory systems.

Bay Leaves Benefits & Uses

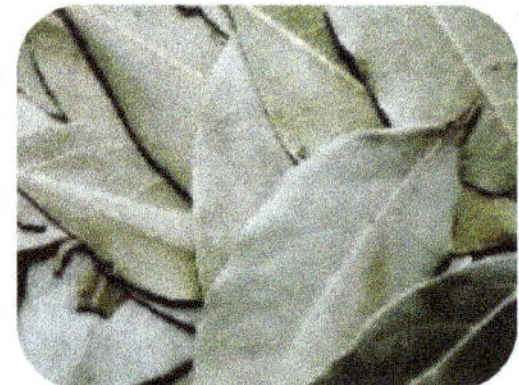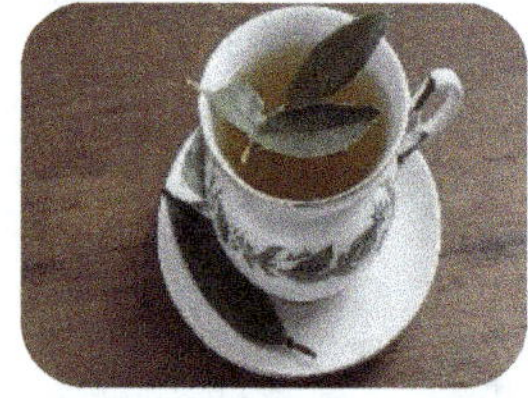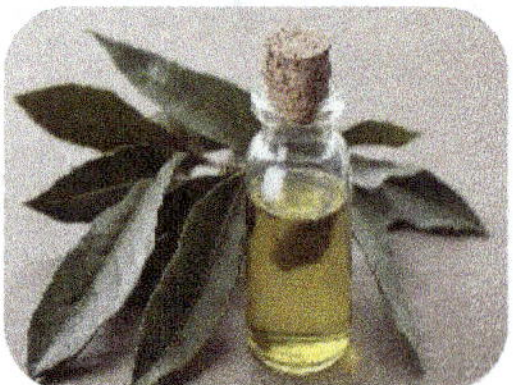

Bay Leaves, Tea & Oil (Design by Freepik)

Bay leaves are rich in nutrients, vitamins, and minerals. Additionally, it is packed with antioxidants, anti-inflammatory, anti-microbial, anti-cancer, and antibacterial components. People with type 2 diabetes may find that consuming bay leaf extract lowers blood sugar and fat levels in the bloodstream and improves diabetes management. It can control cholesterol levels and prevent or treat several cancers, including colorectal, leukemia, and breast cancer.

It supports strong bones, muscles, kidneys, and vision. Furthermore, it strengthens the immune system and promotes cardiovascular and heart health. The flavor of bay leaf is excellent in food. It can be used in many dishes as crushed or whole. Discard whole leaves must be discarded after cooking.

To make bay leaf tea, use 2 tsp ground leaves in two cups of filtered water, boil for 4-5 minutes, then let steep for 5-10 minutes. Strain and enjoy with 1-2 tsp of stevia and other flavorings of your choice.

Bay leaf oil has been used for lower back pain, arthritis, stomach ailments, sore muscles, and sprains.

Lemon Balm

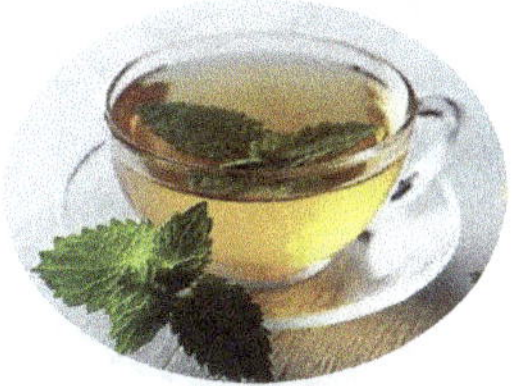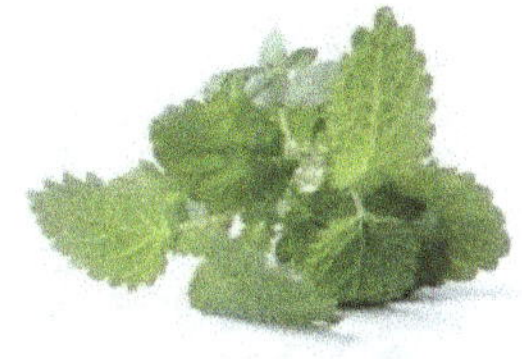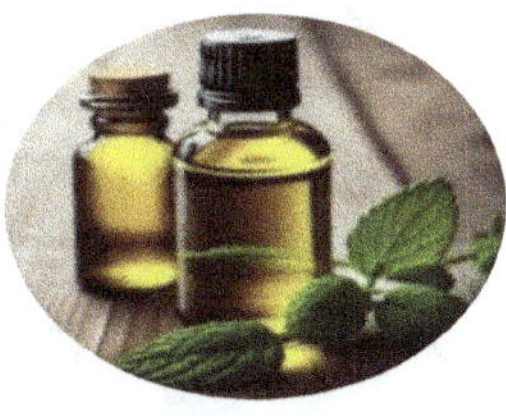

Lemon Balm Tea, Leaves & Oil (Designed by Pixabay & Freepik)

Lemon Balm contains antioxidants, anti-inflammatory, anti-viral, and anti-microbial properties that is another flavorful herb with impressive health advantages for diabetes. Research has shown that extract and oil impact elevated blood sugar by lowering blood sugar levels and protecting against neuropathy and the stress brought on by diabetes. Consistent use can help treat and prevent diabetes.

In addition, lemon balm has properties that may protect against heart, cardiovascular, liver, Alzheimer's, and Parkinson's disease. It may also help with digestion, thyroid issues, and metabolic health. Sprinkle chopped lemon balm or drizzle its oil over salads, fruits, eggs, dips, and smoothies.

Lemon balm tea has all the benefits mentioned earlier, and it also helps with stress, anxiety, mood, relaxation, and sleep. Add chopped lemon balm (or its oil) to smoothies, fruits, salads, eggs, and dips. In addition to the benefits listed above, lemon balm tea and its oil help with anxiety, stress, mood, relaxation, and sleep.

Benefits of Fenugreek

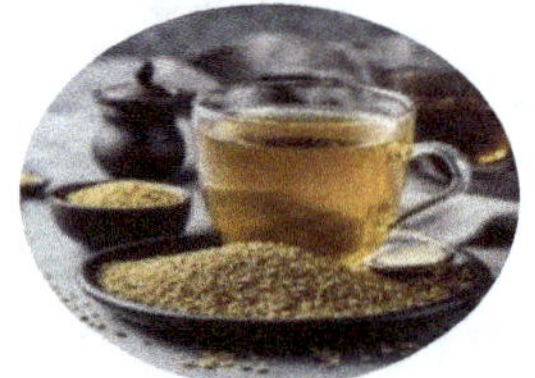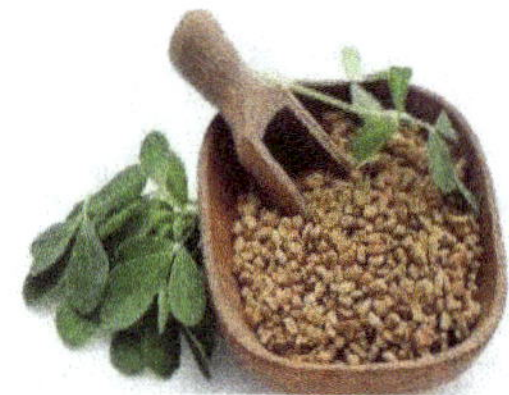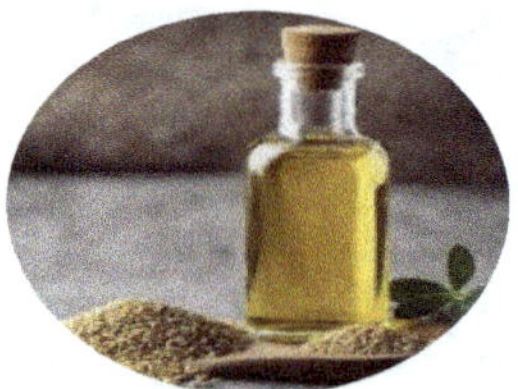

Fenugreek Tea, Leaves & Seeds, & Oil (Designed by Freepik)

Fenugreek is another herb with impressive health benefits. It is packed with vitamins, nutrients, and other compounds that slow sugar transport into the bloodstream, which helps lower blood sugar levels. This herb prevents the spikes and crashes of blood sugar levels and regulates insulin release in the body. Certain cultures eat roasted seeds purely for their natural health benefits for diabetes.

Lower cholesterol, heart disease prevention, immune system stimulation, anti-inflammatory qualities, kidney health promotion, and decreased cancer risk are additional positive health effects. The dried leaves are used as herbs, and the fenugreek seeds are eaten roasted or raw or as a powdered spice. Use the seeds to flavor soups, stews, salads, sauces, and curries. The green leaves can be eaten like microgreens or steamed with garlic and onion for flavor, and the sprouts added to vegetables or salads. Combine by blending the dried leaves with other herbs to season meats, fish, and seafood, or add some nutritious green leaves to the pot. Use the powder to make a cup of tea and use oil in salads and dips.

Benefits of Leek

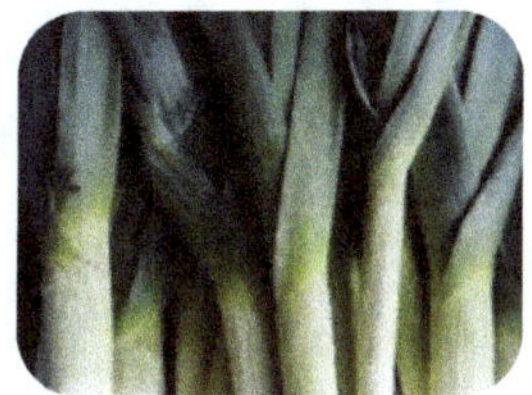

Fresh Leek (Designed by Pixabay)

Leek is a low-glycemic and low-calorie food in the family group of onions and garlic. It contains anti-diabetic, anti-inflammatory, and anti-cancer properties. The plant's compounds, such as allicin, flavonoids (kaempferol), copper, high fiber, and iron, contribute to the following health benefits: regulate blood sugar levels and protect against diabetes, neuropathy, and metallic syndrome.

Consuming leeks may improve insulin sensitivity, where the muscles will absorb glucose to be used for energy rather than being stored in the blood. This protects against high and low blood sugar levels, diabetic neuropathy, and metabolic syndrome and strengthens the diabetic's cardiac function.

It also promotes vision, kidney, brain, and bone health. Regularly consuming leek will prevent cancer/s and stomach ailments, improve metabolism, regenerate damaged cells, prevent heart diseases, lower cholesterol, fight infections, improve digestion, and promote weight gain.

Add chopped leek to beans, soups, salads, and stews. It can be roasted, braised, grilled, steamed, or boiled. Use it as a side dish or mix it with other vegetables.

Fennel's Benefits

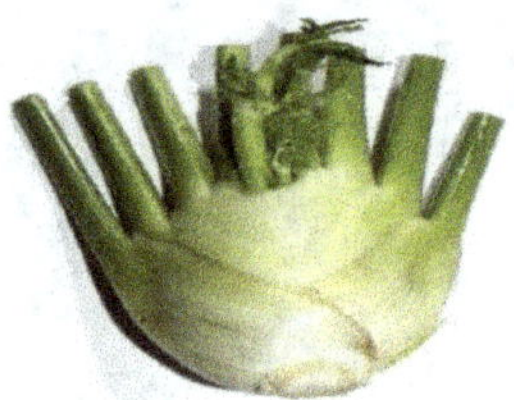

Fennel (Designed by Pixabay)

Fennel seeds and bulbs are packed with antioxidants, minerals, and nutrients. Manganese, one of the minerals in fennel, helps regulate blood sugar levels, treat, and prevent diabetes, and prevent diabetes complications. Additional good news for people with diabetes is that fennel plant compounds reduce high blood pressure and cholesterol levels.

Furthermore, fennel also contains anti-cancer, anti-virus, anti-inflammatory, and antimicrobial properties which is great news for people with diabetes. Regularly consuming fennel may reduce the risks of getting diabetes. Moreover, the properties of fennel may improve brain health, including memory and cognitive skills, strengthen bone density, and promote digestive health.

Fennel is another vegetable that can be eaten raw in salads, with dips and olive oil. It is used in cooking mixed with other vegetables as a single vegetable and in soups. Steamed, grilled, roasted, boiled, or braised fennel is succulent and flavorful. It pairs well with meats, fish, and seafood as a side dish. Roast the fennel seeds and enjoy them as a snack.

Green Onion's/Scallions

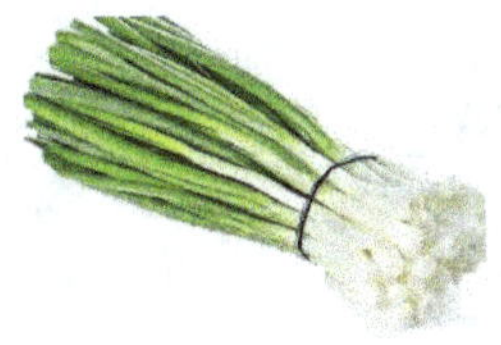

Green Onions/Scallions (Design by Pixabay)

Green onions are rich in antioxidants, anti-cancer, anti-viral, anti-bacterial, and other plant properties. Health benefits for people with diabetes include stimulation and generation of insulin in the pancreas, lower blood sugar levels, and regular consumption may prevent diabetes.

Other benefits for the person with diabetes are lower blood pressure, improved vision, heart, and bone health. It also helps boost the immune system, and aids in digestive and respiratory functions.

Add chopped green onions to soups, stews, sauces, meat dishes, salads, whole wheat pasta dishes, stuffings, vegetables, stir-fry, and curries. Sprinkle chopped onions (or use entire stalk) on meats and fish when baking, roasting, or broiling. I add green onions to many dishes I prepare, even salads. It gives food an exotic flavor and pleasant aroma.

Cilantro Benefits

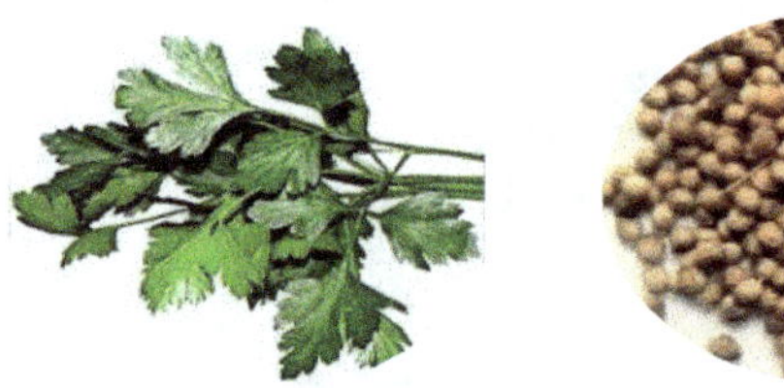

Fresh Cilantro & Cilantro or Coriander Seeds Design by Pixabay)

Cilantro herbs have a pleasant aroma and an exotic flavor that adds a delectable taste to food. It is used in Indian, Mexican, Latino and Caribbean dishes as a seasoning and garnish. Cilantro is rich in antioxidants, minerals and nutrients that can potentially stimulate and produce insulin hormones in the pancreas.

It helps slow the absorption of glucose into the bloodstream, avoid sugar spikes, thus lowering and stabilizing blood sugar levels. People with diabetes will be happy to know that this simple green herb contains more impressive benefits such as protecting eye, kidney, liver, and bone health. It regulates high blood pressure and bad cholesterol levels for a healthy cardiovascular system.

Consuming cilantro also rids the body of toxic metals, prevents cancer and anemia, and fights against Alzheimer's. Cilantro can be used in many dishes, such as sauces, meats, fish, stews, soups, salads, beans, peas, vegetables, salsa, and egg dishes. It is best to wait until the end of cooking to add it for its full flavor and benefits.

Sprinkle chopped cilantro on sandwiches, add it to vegetable and fruit smoothies or salsa, or eat it raw. The seeds are called coriander and can be added to smoothies before blending or boiled for tea. Other options are cilantro pesto, vinaigrette, and oil.

How About Culantro?

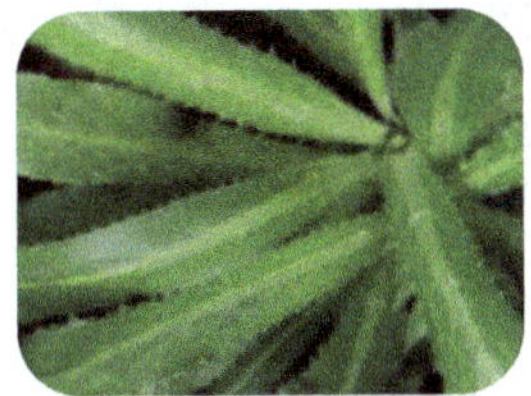

Fresh Culantro (Free Photo Shira's Garden)

Culantro is in the family group as cilantro, an exotic herb not very well known. It has a stronger flavor and gives food a delectable taste. It is known by other names like sawtooth, serrated coriander, recao, fit weed, shado beni, and more. Research has shown that culantro contains compounds that encourage the increase of insulin in the body, which lowers blood glucose levels and reduces diabetes complications. It also promotes liver and brain health and lowers blood pressure.

Culantro is used in many Caribbean, Asian, and Spanish dishes. Use finely chopped culantro in sauces, stews, soups, salads, beans, peas, vegetables, salsa, egg, meat, fish, seafood, and curry dishes. Add culantro to foods towards the end of cooking for its full flavor and benefits or sprinkle raw over dishes. Blend it with cilantro and other green herbs to rub on meats when seasoning, especially curries.

My grandmother grew this herb year-round. She used it abundantly to season and flavor meats, seafood, gravies, sauces, and other foods. The flavor it gives to curried vegetables and meats is to die for. So Yummy!!

Diabetic Benefits of Onions

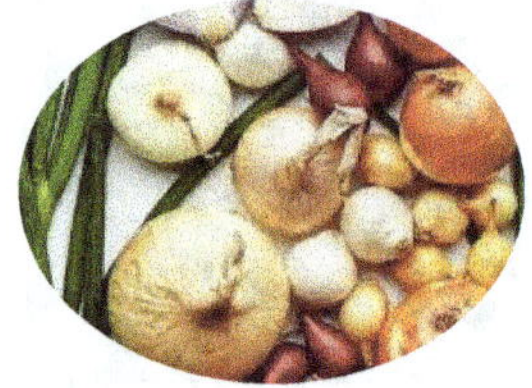

Onion Variety (Design by Pixabay)

Onions, which come in several varieties (yellow, white, shallot, Vidalia, etc.) contribute to good health. They are dense in quercetin, which helps slow the release of blood sugar into the body's cells and muscles, lowers blood sugar levels, and manages diabetes.

More health benefits are they help prevent heart disease and stroke, boost the immune system, have anti-cancer properties, improve memory and cognitive performance, have detoxifying properties, and aid the digestive system.

Sauté onions, add vegetables, meats, eggs, sauces, fish, seafood, stir-fries, and curries. Onions can be grilled, roasted, caramelized, fried, boiled, and served as a side dish. Add raw onions to salads. It goes well caramelized on steaks and other meats. You can include it in stews, sauces, beans, peas, and more dishes, as per your taste.

Chives

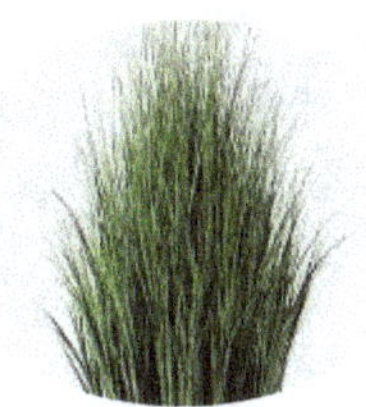

Chive (Design by Freepik)

Chive is related to garlic and onions. It is a thin-leaf herb that grows as a weed in many places, and it is used mainly as a garnish adding a delicate oniony flavor to foods. Chives are incredibly low in calories and rich in antioxidants, minerals, vitamins, and fiber, contributing to health benefits.

While research does not show that it aids diabetes directly, it does show that it lowers blood pressure and cholesterol which helps to decrease the risks of cardiovascular, heart, coronary artery disease and stroke. Consuming chives regularly protects against cancer, improves memory and cognitive performance, treats Alzheimer's, and contributes to eye and bone health.

Add finely chopped chives to stir-fries, stews, soups, sauces, meat dishes, curries, vegetables, salads, and any dish you want. You can garnish omelets, and other egg dishes, meats and more.

Savory's Benefits

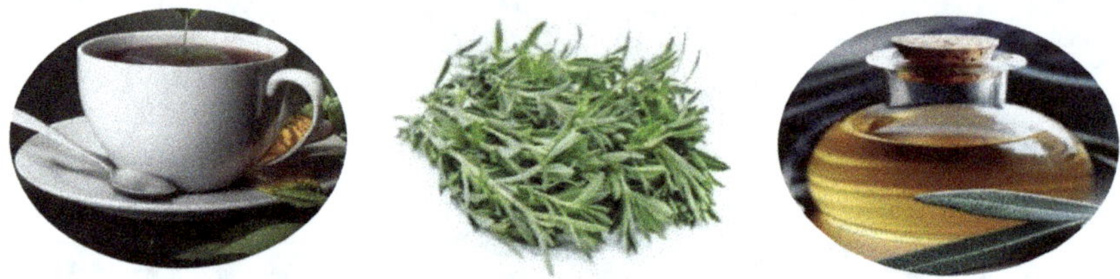

Savory Tea, Leaves & Oil (Designed by Pixabay & Night Cafe)

The savory herb is known in many parts of the world for its potential to treat common health ailments like indigestion, intestinal problems, sore throat, etc. However, recent research and studies have shown that this versatile, tasty herb/plant species has components that offer natural treatment or prevention of diabetes and its complications, cardiovascular disease, Alzheimer's disease, and cancer. Furthermore, its anti-inflammatory, antimicrobial, and antioxidant properties protect against free radical damage that causes chronic illnesses, inflammation, and infections.

Use finely chopped savory to flavor meat, fish, eggs, soup, vegetables, beans, peas, and lentils. Savory tea made from savory herbs is refreshing and helps you unwind at the end of the day. Use the oil in a diffuser as an essential oil or lightly drizzle on salads and dips.

A History Bit of & Herbs & Spices

Herbal medicine in the form of herbs and spices dates back from the early humans, Egypt, Asia, Greece, Rome, the Middle Ages, and the Aztecs to modern-day civilization. The early hunters wrapped meats in leaves from trees, bushes, and brushes and discovered they were flavored and preserved. Purely by trial and error, in ages past, man learned to recognize plants that were good for food, flavor, coloring, healing, and other purposes, as well as those that were poisonous.

Herbs and spices became a trade among countries, from trading post to trading post from one island or town to the next. This eventually resulted in creating wealth for many countries and their people. Through the centuries and generations, herbal plants were used for their medicinal value. Herbs and spice extracts have been (and are still being) used for the healing of ailments and diseases, skincare, haircare, meditation, in temples or monasteries, to make perfumes, as incense, and in baths, for anointing, embalming, to name a few of their purposes.

Medicinal healing came strictly from the roots, stems or stalks, branches, fruit, leaves, and flowers of herbal plants, that is, up until the 19th century when peddlers introduced bottled medicines. Do modern-day medicines come from herbal plants? Are they refined and processed? If so, how efficient are they?

A Little of My History

As a child and well into my teens, I never went to see a doctor or took any pharmaceutical drugs. My grandmother believed in herbal medicine for everything. There was a plant/herb cure for every fever, ache, cramp, bruise, cut, cough, cold, or any other ailment. And every time, it worked. I grew apart from herbal medicine when I became an adult with responsibilities.

For any medical problem, from then on, I saw a doctor and followed their treatment with pharmaceutical drugs. When I was diagnosed with diabetes, I believed that the doctor's treatment would take care of my diabetes, but it did not bring the results I needed. And when it became a grave issue, I decided to transition to all herbal medicine for my diabetes. I am happy to say that within eight months of continuously consuming only organic foods that are low-carb, low glycemic index, have healthy fats, 100% whole wheat or grain (small portions), and other foods that have anti-diabetes properties, along with the herbs, spices, teas, and oils mentioned in this e-book that I saw a change in my blood sugar readings.

My lab results used to show blood sugar levels from 250 and higher and A1C levels from 8 to 10. For the last almost eleven years, I have helped my blood sugar levels to decrease and regulate by eating and drinking all diabetes-friendly food and drinks. I do a little dance every time I check my levels, and they are within normal range before and after meals, and my HbA1c levels remain steady at 6.0 - 6.5. I feel energized, happy, and have won the battle with diabetes.

Garlic's Diabetic Benefits

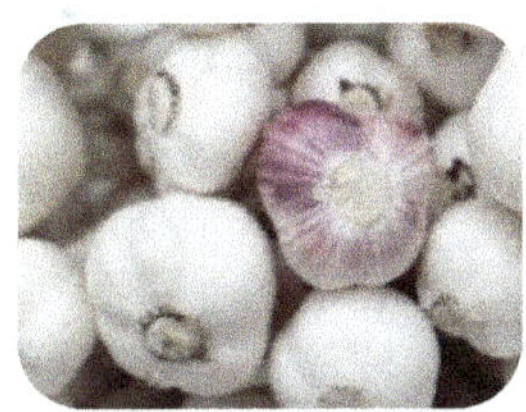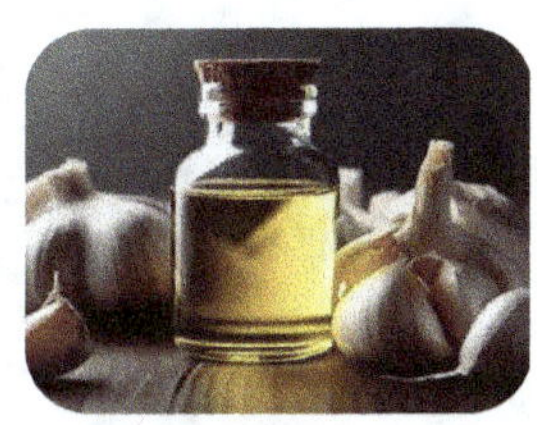

Whole Garlic & Oil (Design by Pixabay & Freepik)

Garlic contains vitamins, nutrients, antioxidants, anti-inflammatory, anti-cancer properties, and phytochemicals (healthy plant compounds) that contribute to a treasure trove of impressive health benefits. Studies have shown that garlic helps treat diabetes by reducing blood glucose levels, high blood pressure, and cholesterol, protecting against neuropathy and the risk of heart and cardiovascular disease, thereby preventing heart attacks and stroke.

Consuming garlic improves brain health, lowers the risk of chronic diseases, strengthens bones, and improves quality of life. It also contributes to a healthy immune system and detoxifies the body.

Use finely chopped or grated garlic in curries, soups, stews, pasta dishes, stir-fries, sauces, vegetables, egg dishes, meats, fish, and seafood.

Garlic oil stimulates circulation, reduces inflammation, optimizes digestion, and contributes to healthy brain function and immune system. It aids with earaches as well. Use garlic oil or pesto in salads, dips, and when sautéing.

Ginger's Benefits

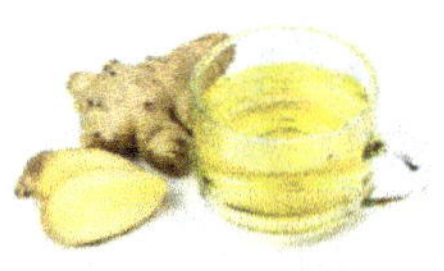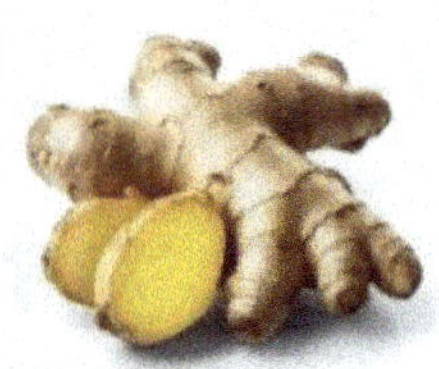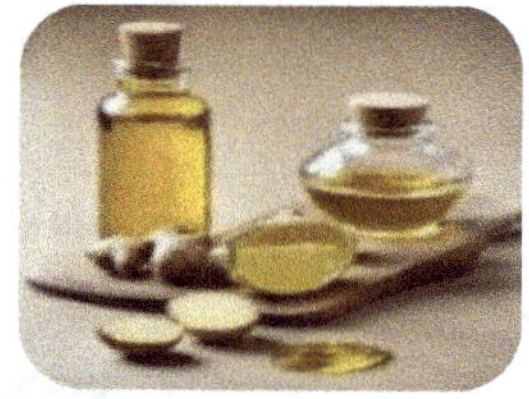

Ginger Tea, Root, & Oil (Designed by Freepik)

Ginger has powerful nutrients, antioxidants, and anti-inflammatory and anti-diabetic properties. Garlic contributes to the reduction and improvement of insulin levels. Research has shown that ginger can dramatically improve HbA1c levels. Garlic has compounds that may prevent chronic illnesses by reducing oxidative stress.

Other impressive benefits include protection against diabetic complications, lower cholesterol, and improved brain functions, which may prevent Alzheimer's and protect against cancer, stomach problems, osteoarthritis, and infections.

Grated ginger is excellent as a seasoning agent. Add it to marinades, stews, curries, soups, sauces, vegetables, and stir-fries. Delicious! Blend it with homemade juices, vegetables, or green smoothies. Brew it for tea or make ginger beer (non-alcoholic) or a cake.

Ginger oil is used for aromatherapy. I embrace the health benefits of ginger; it is a super healthy spice that I include in my daily diet.

Turmeric's Diabetic Benefits

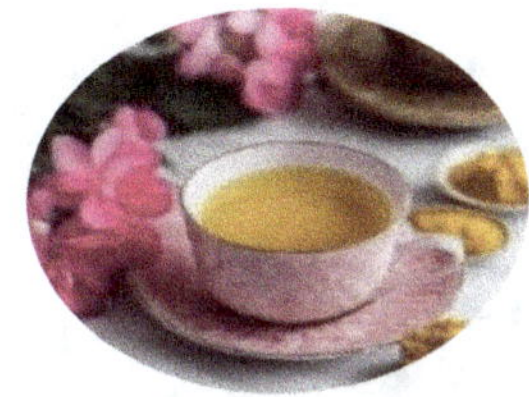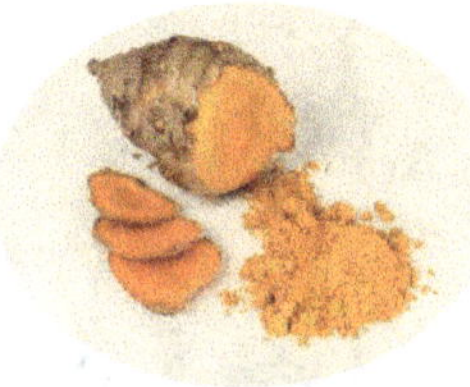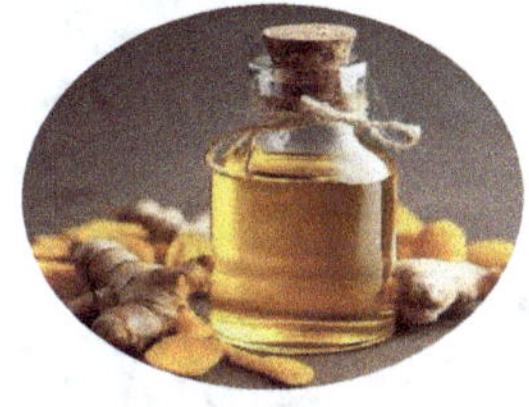

Turmeric Tea, Spice & Oil (Designed by Pixabay & Freepik)

Turmeric plant compounds hold many impressive health benefits. Its antioxidants and anti-inflammatory properties may play a role in helping to treat and fight against and may prevent diabetes. Certain cultures believe that it is an excellent treatment for diabetes.

More health benefits include reduced risks of neuropathy, enhanced heart, liver, and brain health. It can also decrease the risks of cancer, tumors, strengthen the immune system, and promote digestive health.

Turmeric is best when used in pure form. Add a small amount (1/2 tsp) to stews, sauces, soups, veggies, eggs, and meat dishes. I mix a small amount, about ½ teaspoon, in warm milk with stevia and a dash of cinnamon for a healthy drink. Turmeric oil is used primarily for skin health.

Health Benefits of Flaxseeds

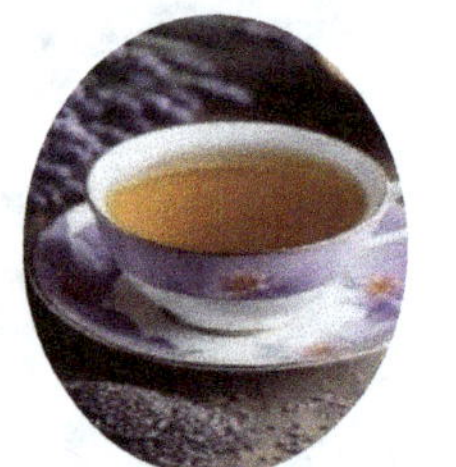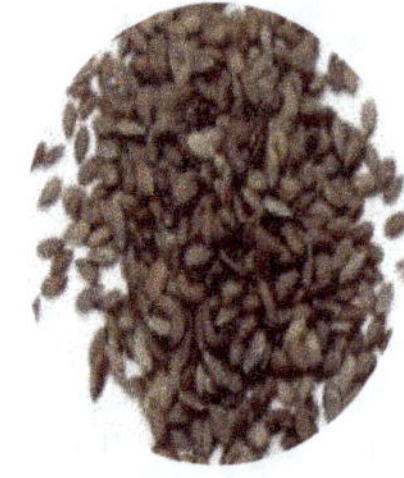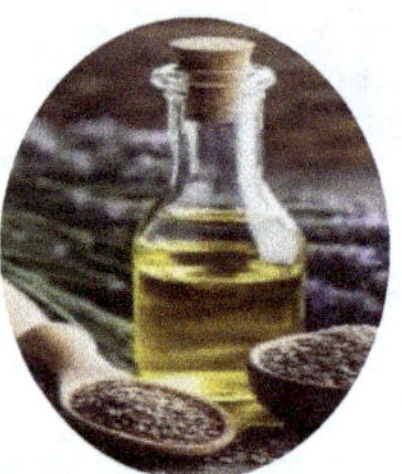

Flax Seeds, Tea & Oil (Designed by Pixabay & Freepik)

Studies with flaxseed have shown that it stimulates insulin secretions, which reduces blood sugar and HbA1c levels. It contains antioxidants, minerals, proteins, and anti-inflammatory compounds that may contribute to heart, liver, bone, brain, kidney, and digestive health. Studies also show that flaxseed reduces the risk of lung and breast cancer, boosts immune system health, and promotes weight loss.

Flaxseed can be eaten raw, roasted, or ground. Begin with a pinch of grounded flaxseed and gradually increase to 1-2 tbsp a day when your body adjusts. Add it to hot or cold cereal, fruit, and yogurt. Add raw or roasted seeds to salads or smoothies.

Use flax flour to make pancakes, bread, cakes, pies, or muffins. Use it as a binder instead of eggs in meatloaf and baked macaroni.

The tea offers cardiovascular health, lower blood sugar, and anticancer properties. Use the oil in salads, dips, and sauces. It is also healthy for skin and hair.

Health Benefits of Cinnamon

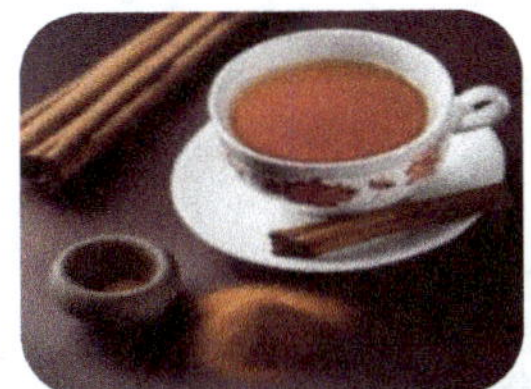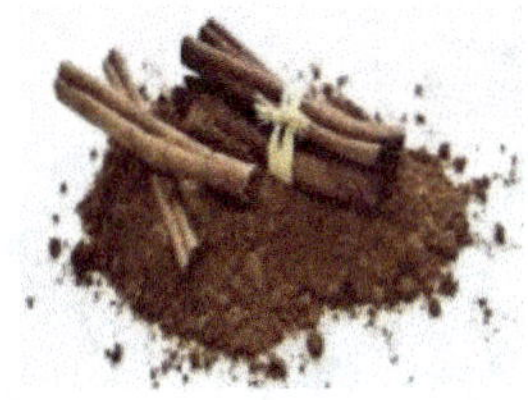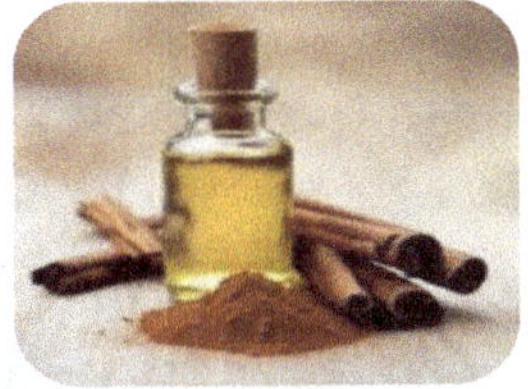

Cinnamon Tea, Spice, & Oil (Designed by Freepik)

Cinnamon is a power spice. The powerful polyphenol antioxidants that have anti-inflammatory properties lower the risks of many diseases. Studies have proven that cinnamon drastically reduces insulin resistance. It increases insulin sensitivity, acts on cells that mimic insulin, slows the absorption of sugar into the bloodstream, and can bring sugar levels to normal. More great benefits include heart, cardiovascular, neurodegenerative (brain) health and prevention and treatment of cancer. Its anti-viral and anti-bacterial properties help prevent viruses.

Sprinkle cinnamon over hot or cold cereals, cooked oatmeal, yogurts, fruits, shakes, smoothies, and warm milk. When baking, add it to cakes, muffins, pies, pancakes, bread, and cookies. Use cinnamon in meats, sweet potato dishes, stews, sauces, or any food you want. Brew it as tea with a mint leaf or a bit of ginger; it is delicious and healthy. Sweeten with stevia. Cinnamon oil can be used in a diffuser mixed with a carrier oil for massages, as a bath oil, to scent your home, or to stimulate the senses.

Nutmeg's Benefits

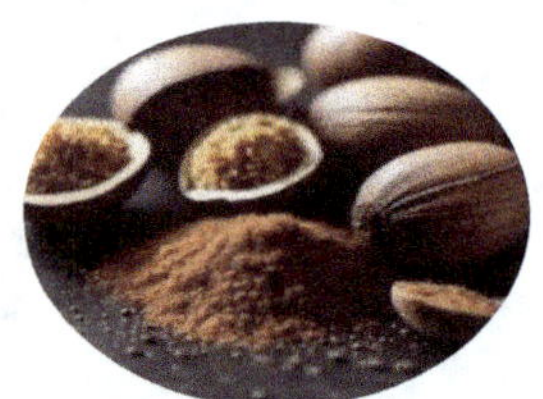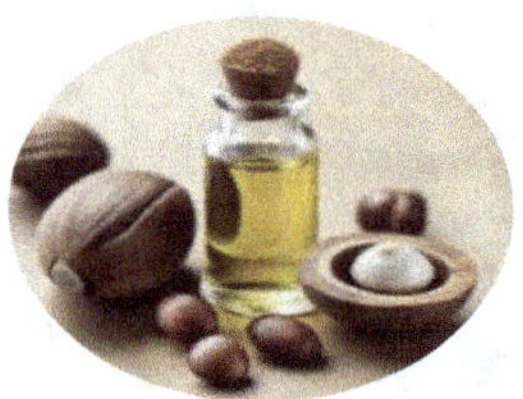

Whole & Ground Nutmeg & Oil (Designed by Freepik)

Nutmeg may help reduce blood sugar levels and stimulate insulin secretions in the pancreas. The plant's compounds include antioxidants, nutrients, and anti-inflammatory agents. These have the potential to fight against diabetes, heart disease and cancer. In addition to protecting against Alzheimer's disease, consuming nutmeg improves blood circulation, boosts immune health, promotes digestion, detoxifies the body, and prevents and fights bacteria.

Sprinkle a pinch or two of nutmeg over hot or cold cereals on yogurts, fruits, shakes, smoothies, eggs, veggies, and warm milk. When baking, add it to cakes, muffins, pies, pancakes, bread, and cookies. Add a pinch or two to soups, curries, stews, cauliflower, cabbage, or carrots.

Mix a pinch or two in 8 oz (about 236.59 ml) of water and drink each day or drink a warm cup of nutmeg tea before bed. Add grated nutmeg to a cup of warm milk. Drizzle oil on fruit, yogurts, and salads.

Benefits In Cloves

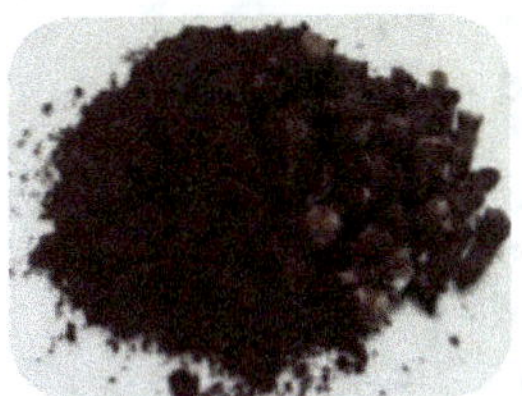 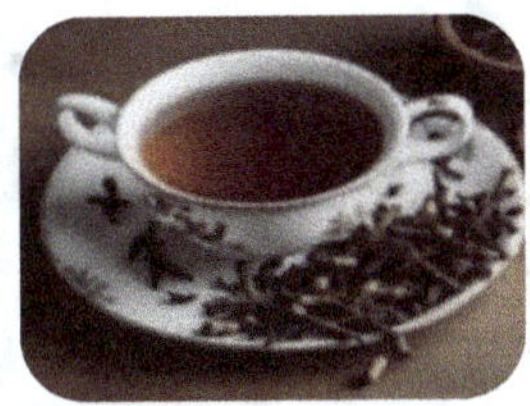 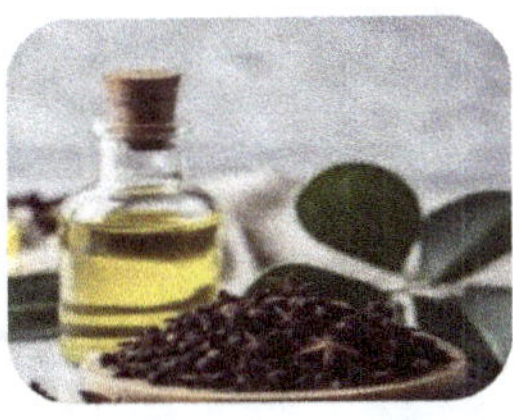

Whole & Ground Cloves (Design by Pixabay) Clove Tea & Oil (Designed by Freepik)

The plant properties in cloves have the potential to mimic, stimulate and produce insulin secretions in the pancreas. Consuming cloves in certain foods will help regulate blood sugar levels. Clove, included with a plant-based diet, can benefit people with diabetes. It is rich in antioxidants, which are ideal for protecting vital organs. Its nutrients preserve and improve liver, bone, digestive, and immune health. It also promotes blood circulation, relieves pain, and helps protect against neuropathy.

Add ground clove to cakes, pies, squash, and pumpkin dishes. Sprinkle over desserts, warm milk, smoothies, and hot or cold cereal. Add 1/8 teaspoon to stews, sauces, beans, chili, and soups. Stick whole cloves on whole hams before baking and rub crushed or ground cloves on meats as part of the seasoning.

Clove tea also contributes to the health mentioned earlier benefits. Clove oil contains analgesic, anti-inflammatory, and antimicrobial and has been used as a traditional medicine for pain, toothaches, and therapeutic applications.

Paprika's Diabetic Benefits

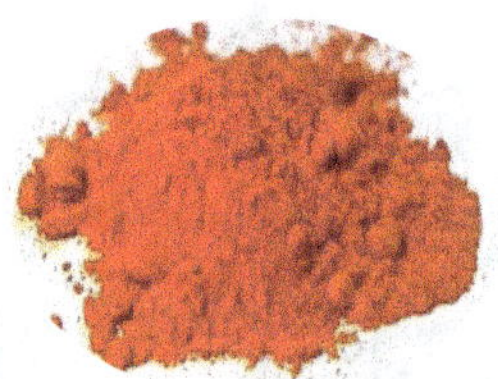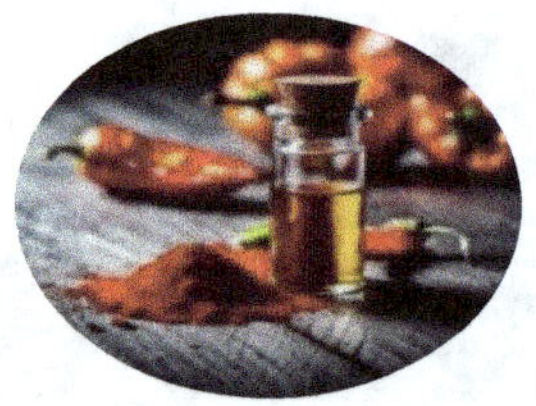

Paprika Spice (Design by Pixabay) Paprika Oil (Designed by Freepik)

Paprika is a spice made from certain peppers rich in antioxidants, minerals, vitamins, and anti-inflammatory properties that host an array of health benefits. One component called capsaicin may influence genes and inhibit enzymes that break down sugar, thus controlling blood levels, preventing sugar spikes, improving insulin sensitivity, and helping manage diabetes.

It may help lower cholesterol, ease diabetic neuropathy pain, promote eye and vision health, boost the immune system, and prevent nerve damage and cell damage due to chronic illnesses, including heart disease and cancer.

Sprinkle paprika on all salads, eggs, meat dishes, sandwiches, and fish. Paprika oil is excellent for grilling, seasoning meats, and vegetables, sauteing, and marinating. Drizzle over salads, soups, and stews.

Health Benefits in Cumin

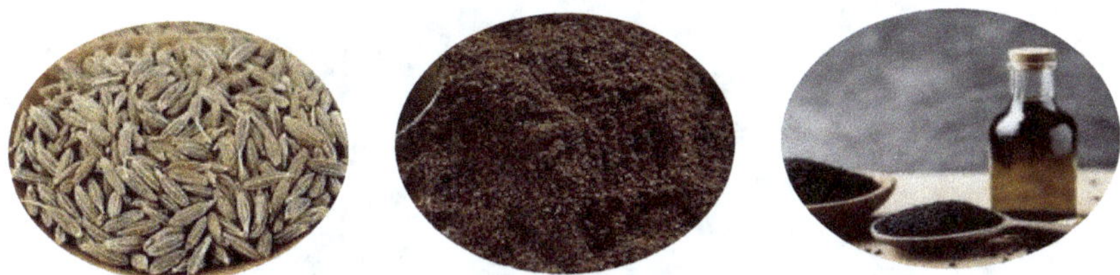

Cumin Seeds & Ground Cumin & Oil (Design by Pixabay & Freepik)

Cumin is a spice that is rich in plant compounds such as antioxidants, anti-inflammatory, antibiotics antibacterial, antifungal, iron, and minerals, which support healthy blood sugar levels. It treats and helps prevent the long-term complications of diabetes and possibly prevent diabetes itself.

Additional health benefits include protection against neuropathy, kidney, heart, brain, and eye disease. Consuming cumin will also help promote healthy blood vessels, lower cholesterol levels, reduce the risks of cancer and protect against food-borne illnesses.

Add a small amount of ground-roasted cumin to curries, stews, sauces, beans, chili, and soups. Sprinkle whole roasted seeds on salads and vegetables. Include ground-roasted cumin in seasonings or marinades for all meats, fish, and seafood. Cumin oil improves brain functions and enhances overall health.

Cardamon Spice

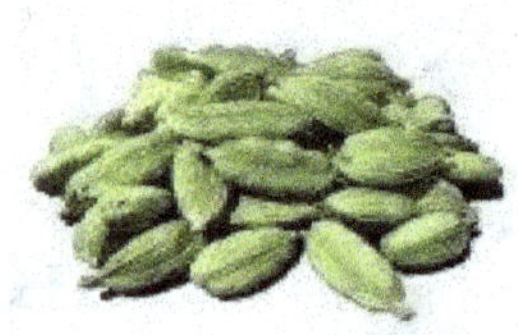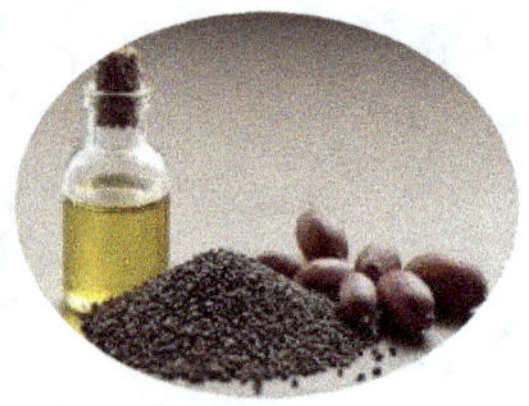

Cardamon Seeds & Oil (Design by Freepik)

Cardamon spice has plant properties that hold a variety of health benefits. It is rich in antioxidants, anti-inflammatory, certain enzymes, diuretic, and other compounds that may have the potential to lower blood sugar levels in people with high blood glucose. Additionally, consuming cardamon spice may reduce blood pressure, cholesterol, triglyceride, and diabetes stress that leads to anxiety, depression and mood disorders which are markers for a healthy cardiovascular system.

Furthermore, the plant's compounds may protect against inflammation in the body which can prevent chronic illnesses, liver problems, cancers, and tumors. More health benefits include improved digestive health, healthy lungs, and oral health. Using cardamon essential oil in a diffuser can improve breathing, prevent certain bacterial strains, help with asthma, and weight loss.

Chamomile Tea & Oil

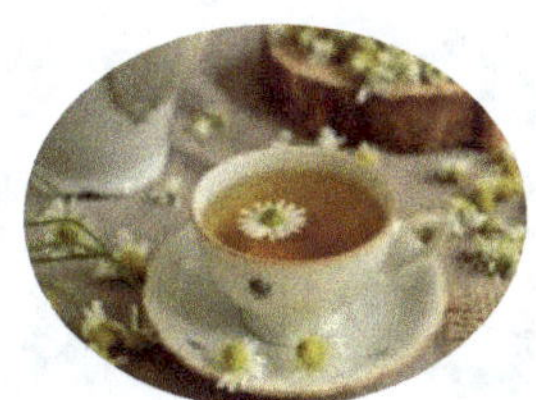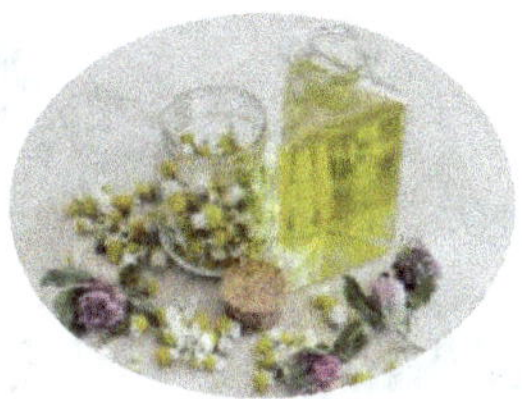

Chamomile Tea & Oil (Design by Pixabay)

Chamomile is a worldwide popular herb used for tea. It has antioxidants, antibacterial, anti-inflammatory, anti-cancer and antiseptic properties, vitamins, minerals, and nutrients that significantly benefit the human body. Studies with chamomile tea have shown that it may prevent high blood sugar levels, help manage diabetes and reduce the long-term risks of diabetes. Additionally, chamomile tea may improve heart and cardiovascular systems and bone health, boost the immune system, protect against cancer, prevent stress and anxiety, and promote sleep. 1-2 cups a day will yield results.

Chamomile oil has become popular throughout the modern age. It is aromatherapy used in a diffuser in a well-ventilated room. Before using it on the skin it must be diluted with a carrier oil of your choice. Mix it with lotion, and use it as a massage oil, in your bath, or on a hot compress to apply to pain areas.

Dandelion's Benefits

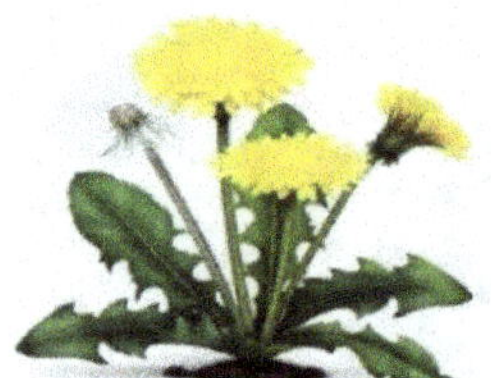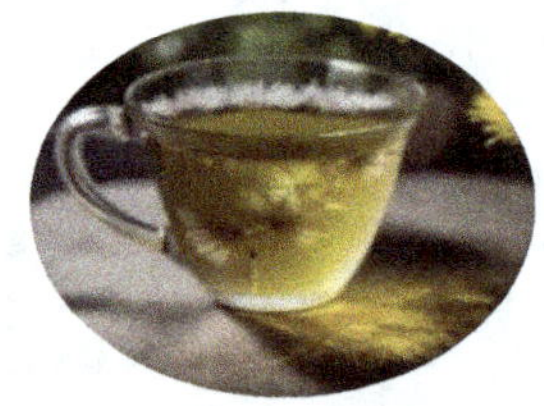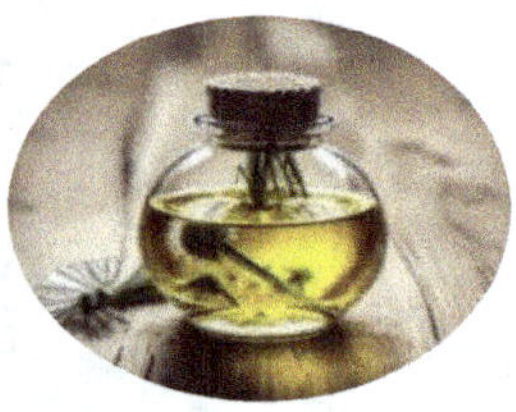

Dandelion Weed/Plant, Tea & Oil (Designed by Freepik)

The entire dandelion plant is packed with nutritional value. Healthy compounds include antioxidants, anti-inflammatory, and anti-bacterial properties, fiber, and other minerals and vitamins. Research has shown evidence that the compounds from the dandelion root can stimulate insulin production from the pancreas and promote the absorption of sugar into the cells and muscle tissues. This results in improved insulin sensitivity and lower blood sugar and HbA1c levels.

Dandelion is high in potassium, an electrolyte and mineral, contributing to a regular heartbeat. Some cultures use dandelion tea to stabilize and control blood sugar. Because it reduces inflammation and produces insulin, they regard it as a natural cure for diabetes and diabetes prevention. More benefits may include lower blood pressure and cholesterol, a healthier heart and cardiovascular system, proper kidney functions, improved blood circulation, the prevention of cancer, liver disease, digestive disorders, chronic illnesses due to inflammation, oxidative stress, and free radical damage, boost the immune system, and detoxify the body.

Taking diabetes medications and drinking dandelion tea can cause blood sugar levels to drop drastically. Seek advice. You must always drink dandelion tea sparingly. Use dandelion virgin oil as a massage oil to remove tension caused by stress in the muscle tissues. It relieves back and neck aches, sore muscles, and joint pain.

Mauby Bark Drink Benefits

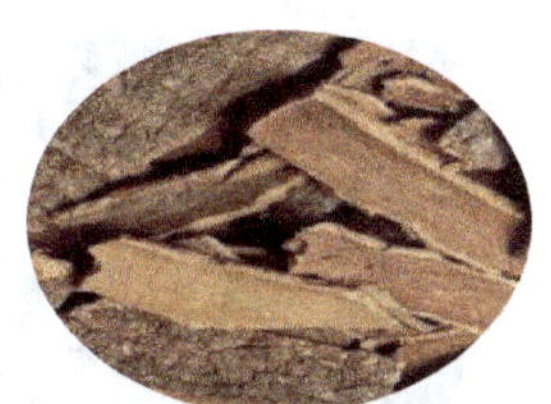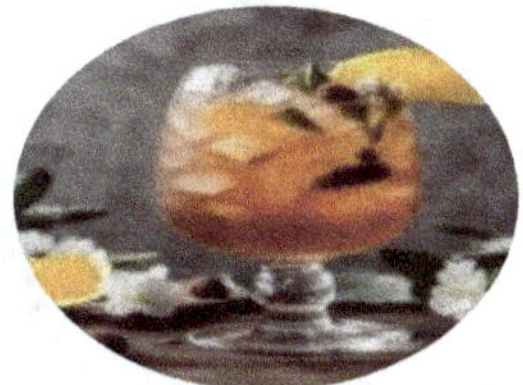

Mauby Bark & Drink (Designed by Freepik)

Mauby bark used to be a strictly Caribbean drink, but it has become known and popular in many other places worldwide. This drink is highly nutritious and is rich in plant properties that contain super health advantages. These include regulating blood glucose levels, increasing insulin sensitivity, stronger immune system, improved blood pressure and cholesterol levels, helping relieve arthritis and joint pain, and removal of toxins in the blood.

Drinking mauby bark tea also reduces the risk of cancers and Alzheimer's, breaks down, and prevents blood clots. It also aids with depression, stress, and anxiety and improves digestive health.

To make mauby bark from concentrate: use five cups of filtered water, 10-15 pieces of mauby bark, add two sticks of cinnamon, 6-8 cloves and 8-10 anise seeds, and ½ teaspoon of grated nutmeg. Boil for 5-7 minutes, cover, and let steep for about 12 hours. When ready to drink, remove and discard ingredients, mix one cup of concentrate with two cups filtered water, and sweeten with (not sugar) but a sweetener like stevia or monk fruit.

Mauby is my favorite drink. I grew up drinking this beverage and had forgotten about it for years until I found it again in an international supermarket in 2017. I learned about mauby bark's health benefits when I began researching teas and drinks that are diabetes friendly.

Black Tea's Benefits

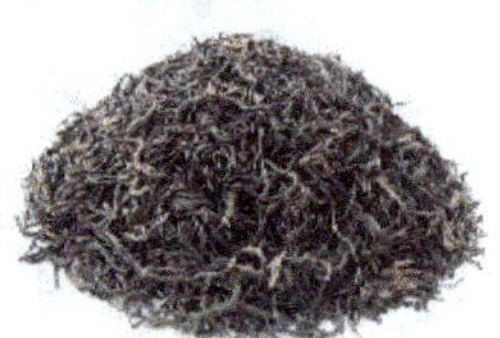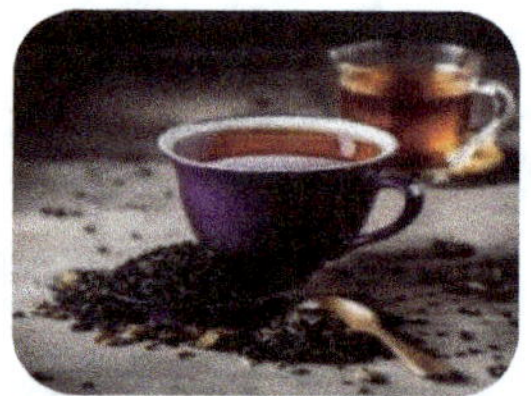

Black Tea (Design by Pixabay & Freepik)

There are several varieties and names of black tea. Several studies with black tea show that it contains plant properties that help to increase insulin activity and improve the use of insulin in the body. Other results found that black tea lowered and regulated blood sugar levels and improved the metabolism of sugar in the body.

It also contributes to heart and brain health, prevents strokes, and has anti-cancer properties. Other health advantages include:

Reduced blood pressure and cholesterol levels.

Protecting against cancer risks.

Stimulating kidney functions.

Hydrating the body.

Improving cognitive functions.

Promoting digestive health.

Add one teaspoon of black tea leaves to eight ounces of boiling filtered water, cover, and let steep for 3-5 minutes, no more than 5 minutes, strain, and add lemon or sweeten (not sugar) to your taste. Enjoy.

Green Tea Benefits

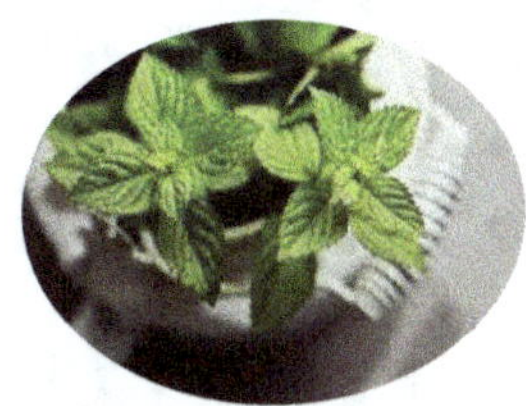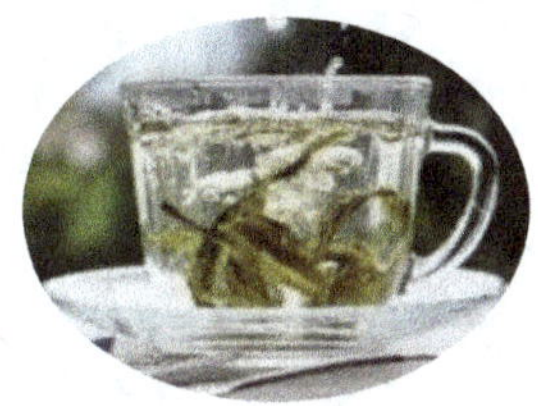

Green Leaf Tea (Design by Pixabay)

The plant compounds in green tea leaves contain several nutritional health benefits. There are several types of green tea which may slow sugar production and absorption in the bloodstream. This process may regulate and maintain blood sugar and HbA1c levels.

Green tea produces insulin by stimulating pancreatic functions and protecting its beta cells from damage and prevent diabetic complications. It is also beneficial for heart and cardiovascular health. Green tea oil reduces inflammation disorders, fights skin aging, softens and moisturizes the skin, and promotes collagen synthesis.

To make green tea, bring two cups of filtered water to a boil, add two teaspoons of fresh or dried green tea leaves, and stir; let the mixture steep for 2-3 minutes, strain, and add flavoring such as a few drops of lemon or sweetened stevia.

Rooibos Tea Benefits

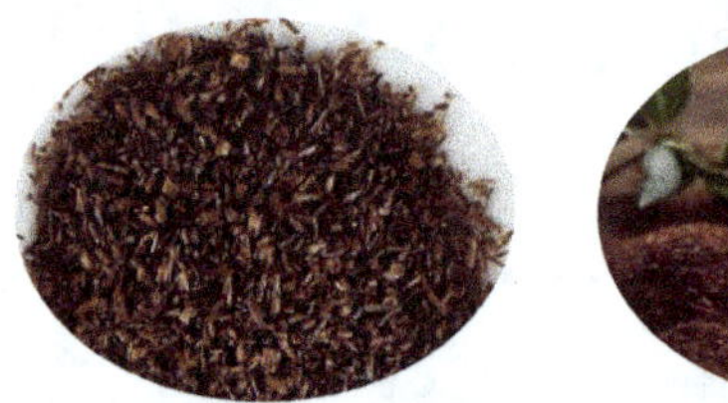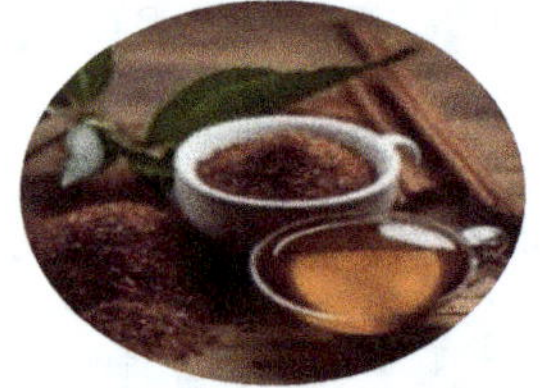

Rooibos Tea (Designed by Pixabay & Freepik)

Rooibos or red bush tea helps cells slowly absorb blood sugar into the bloodstream, thus lowering blood sugar levels. Consuming rooibos tea daily improves insulin sensitivity and reduces the risk of diabetes. It may also prevent heart, bone, and digestive diseases. Other health advantages include protection from cell damage and cancers, and enhanced kidney and brain health.

Rooibos tea has calming effects for that end-of-the-day unwind. Before you consume rooibos tea, please seek professional advice if you are not familiar with rooibos tea.

To make a perfect cup of rooibos tea, use eight ounces of filtered water and one teaspoon of loose-leaf rooibos tea. Have loose-leaf tea ready in a cup, bring water to a rolling rapid boil, then pour water into the cup and let it steep for 5-7 minutes, strain, add sweet, and enjoy.

Oolong Tea Benefits

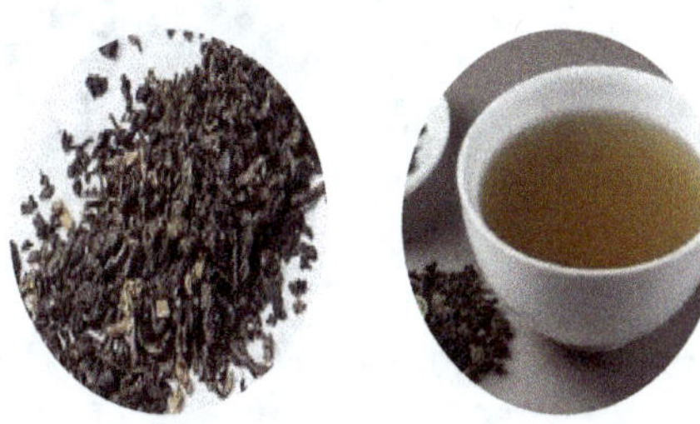

Oolong Tea (Designed by Freepik)

Oolong (there are several types) is rich in polyphenols; potent antioxidants proven to regulate blood sugar levels and even prevent diabetes. Consuming oolong tea may also reduce the risks of heart and cardiovascular disease and stroke and lower blood pressure and cholesterol levels. It may also boost brain and immune health, cognitive performance, and mental alertness and prevent Parkinson's disease. Daily oolong tea may reduce cancer risk, improve bone density and digestive and colon health, and enhance dental health, sleep, and energy. Oolong tea also promotes weight loss.

To make oolong tea, bring 6 ounces of pure filtered water to a rapid boil, add two tablespoons of fresh or dried loose-leaf oolong tea in a teacup, pour water into the cup, cover, and let steep for 2-5 minutes, depending on the strength you want your tea (taste every minute for perfection), strain, add a slice of lemon and enjoy. I add ½ of a stevia leaf while steeping a pinch of nutmeg and cinnamon. You can also drink oolong tea chilled with ice and a slice of fruit such as pear, peach, mango, or whatever you choose.

Benefits in Mint Tea

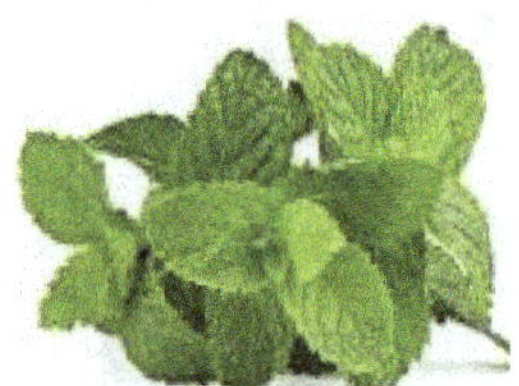 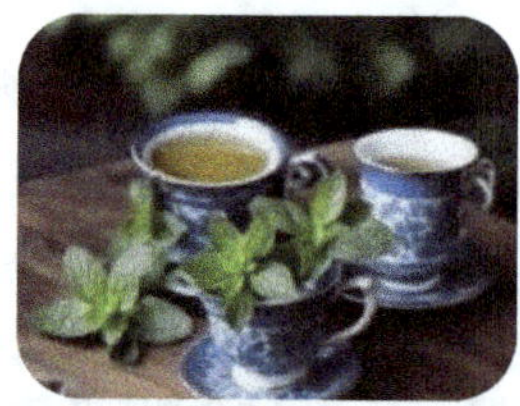

Peppermint Leaf & Tea (Designed by Pixabay & Freepik)

There are several varieties of mint tea, such as peppermint, orange mint, spearmint, Egyptian mint, lavender mint, basil mint, etc., and these mint teas are rich in antioxidants named polyphenols and flavonoids that have a positive impact on diabetes. These plant compounds help reduce blood glucose levels by improving insulin secretions in the body. Polyphenols may target cells that do not respond to insulin, do their job to activate those cells, and make them more receptive. However, mint tea may not be ideal for those taking diabetes medication, seek your doctor's advice. Other benefits include cardiovascular and metabolic health.

Drinking mint tea may also hydrate the blood, protect the liver and kidneys (but not those with kidney stones), enhance brain functions, help stomach disorders, strengthen the immune system, and improve digestion. Mint tea's antibacterial properties will help with headaches, allergies, colds and flu, clogged airways, and improve concentration.

To make mint tea, bring to a rapid boil 2 cups of filtered water, add about 13-15 fresh mint leaves of your choice, turn off the heat, cover, and let steep for 3-5 minutes or a little longer, but no more than 8 minutes, strain, add flavoring of your choice (never sugar) and enjoy. You can also enjoy mint tea chilled with ice.

Ginseng Tea

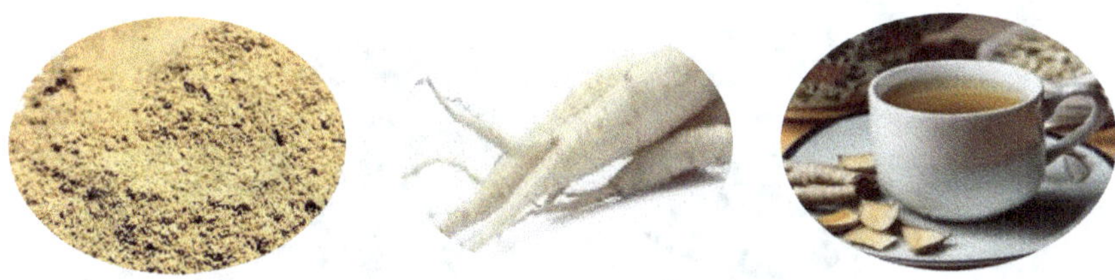

Ginseng Root, Powder & Tea (Designed by Pixabay & Freepik)

Studies have shown that consuming both American and Asian ginseng tea, 2-3 grams a day, helped normalize blood sugar levels and improve hemoglobin A1c in diabetic patients. Ginseng plays a role in controlling the pancreas's defective response to insulin by helping to stimulate and process any insulin in the cells and improving insulin sensitivity and production. Ginseng's antioxidants help reduce free radicals in the cells of people with diabetes and reduce the risks of chronic illnesses and diabetes complications.

More substances in ginseng help prevent sugar spikes after meals, contribute to heart and cardiovascular health (and may even treat diseases), boost the immune system, reduce oxidative stress in the body, improve cognitive and mental functions, protect against cancers, increase energy level, enhance blood circulation, boost metabolism, burn fat, promote restful sleep, and may help with depression, and anxiety.

To make American or some Asian ginseng tea, boil one cup of filtered water, add 1-2 teaspoons of rinsed and thoroughly cleaned ginseng root, reduce heat, and simmer for 15-20 minutes. Strain and add flavoring to your taste and desire (I usually use one half to one stevia leaf from my stevia plant to sweeten my tea and flavor it with lemon. Drink sparingly.

Mulberry Leaf Tea

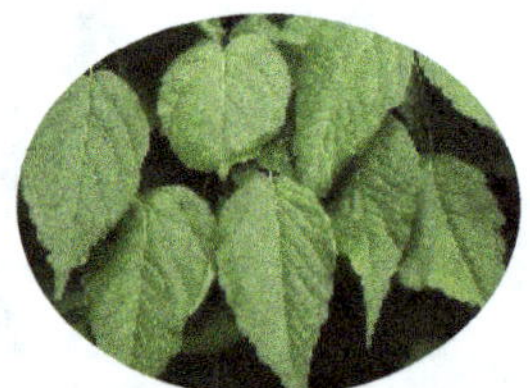 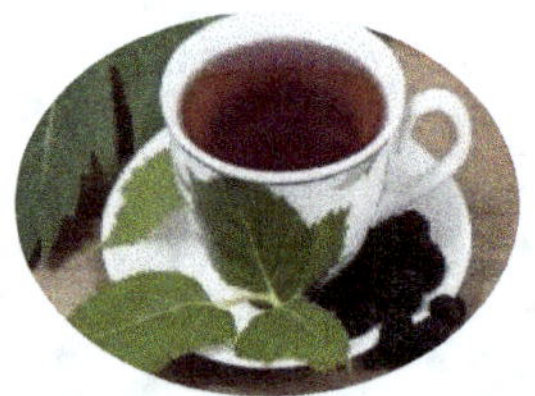

Mulberry Leaves & Tea (Design by Pixabay and Freepik)

Mulberry leaves are highly nutritious. They are rich in antioxidants, anti-inflammatory properties, minerals, and vitamins. Studies have shown that consuming mulberry tea significantly helped in slowing the absorption of sugar into the bloodstream, lowering blood sugar, and improving insulin levels in the pancreas.

In addition, it may regulate blood pressure and cholesterol levels, decrease inflammation, reduce the risks of cell damage, and prevent the arteries from accumulating plaque (atherosclerosis) which leads to heart disease. Furthermore, mulberry leaf tea may prevent or fight against certain cancers, such as liver and cervical cancer. It protects and reduces liver inflammation and damage and may also promote weight loss. Warning: Please consult your doctor before consuming mulberry tea. Follow instructions well.

Moringa Leaf Tea

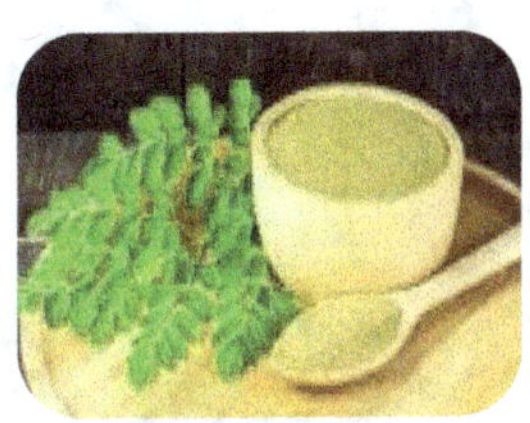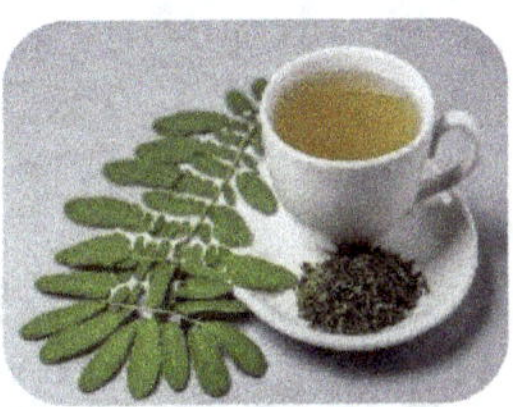

Moringa Leaves, Powder & Tea (Design by Pixabay & Freepik)

From leaves to roots, the moringa plant has healing powers and has traditionally been used for centuries for its medicinal benefits. The plant is packed with antioxidants, anti-inflammatory and anti-cancer properties, vitamins, and important minerals, including potassium, calcium, protein, and amino acids.

These compounds can benefit people with diabetes because studies have shown that it contains proteins and chemicals that can are like insulin thus helping to slow the absorption of sugar into the bloodstream, improve insulin levels, and help control diabetes. Additional health benefits may include the lowering of blood pressure and cholesterol, fat reduction in the blood, stronger immune system, protecting body cells against damage due to free radicals, preventing brain inflammation and improving memory and cognitive skills, treat and keep pancreatic cancer and other cancers at bay, detoxify the body and boost energy levels, and help with arthritis swelling and pain.

Warning: Ask your healthcare provider for advice about this product before consuming moringa tea.

Aloe Vera Benefits

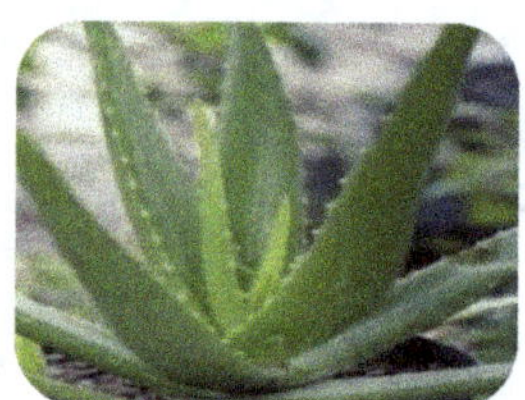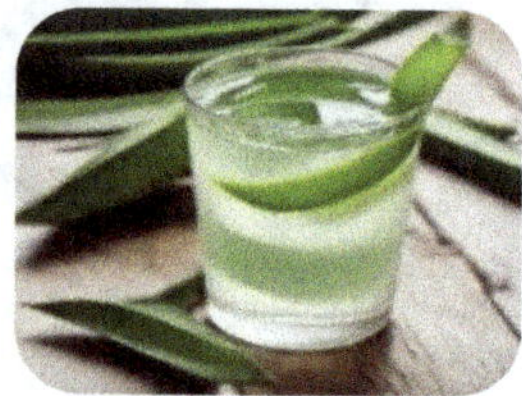

Aloe Vera Plant & Juice (Design by Pixabay & Freepik)

Recent studies suggest that aloe vera's anti-inflammatory properties and antioxidants can help people with diabetes effectively achieve diabetes management. It improves glucose and HbA1c levels. It is well-known for its healing powers and can regulate blood sugar levels and restrict the progression of diabetes. It may even be crucial to the prevention of diabetes. In addition, it has the potential to improve the health of the pancreas's cells and those responsible for insulin production, thus increasing the production of insulin levels.

More benefits include improved eye health, regulated blood pressure, lower cholesterol levels, liver disease, and reduced risks of cancers, heart diseases, and diabetes. It is also suitable for reducing belly fat, improving oral health, promoting digestive health, hydrated and glowing skin, and detoxifying the body and liver. Aloe vera juice is safe to consume because it has very little side effects. However, aloe vera juice must be drunk in moderation and on an empty stomach for full results. However, consult your doctor before drinking aloe vera juice.

To make aloe vera juice, slice about 2 inches off each end of a leaf of aloe vera, let it stand upright in a container to drain the yellow aloe latex for an hour, have a bowl with 1 cup of filtered water and one tablespoon white vinegar mixture ready, then slice off the thorny edges on both sides, using gloves peel off the top part of the leaf, use a large spoon to scoop off the aloe gel from bottom to top, then place the gel in the bowl and rinse off the remaining yellow sticky aloe latex, make sure that only the white gel remains, place in a blender, add 2 cups water, sweetener like stevia to your taste, and the juice from 2 lemons or limes. Other options are the juice from other fresh fruits of your choice, for example, mango, strawberry, etc., cut, blended, and strained (take note of the natural sweetness in fruits.)

I remember my grandmother giving me pieces of aloe vera gel (very bitter) at least twice a week (I was 12 years old and had begun having my monthly periods), and I dared not say no to her, so when she placed it on my tongue, I held my breath, closed my mind, and swallowed it. Ugh!! I never understood then why she did that, but eventually, I found out that, according to her, it was a precaution against pregnancy. I rediscovered and researched the potential health benefits of aloe vera, and I was surprised about the actual health advantages of this plant for diabetes.

Mango Leaf Benefits

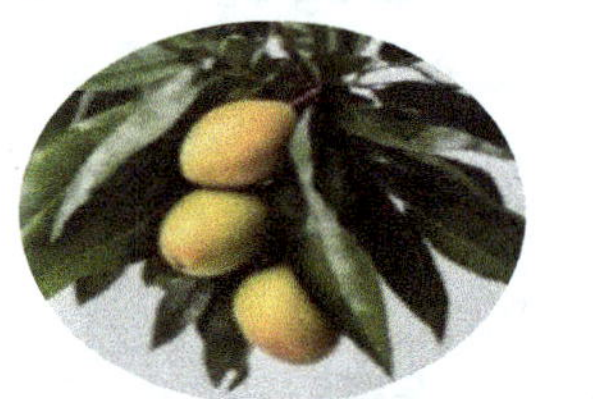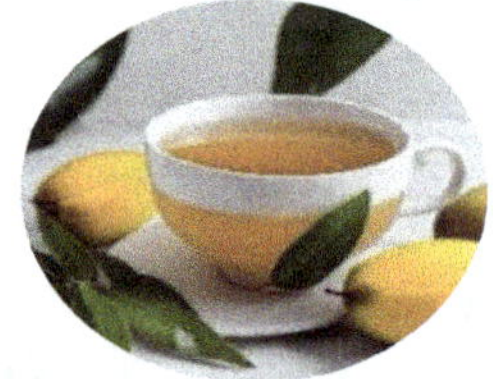

Mango Leaves & Tea (Designed by Freepik)

Mango leaves are rich in antioxidants, anti-bacterial, anti-microbial, anti-inflammatory properties, vitamins, and other compounds that protect against diseases and fight inflammation. Mango leaf tea may treat the early signs of diabetes, slow the progression of diabetes, and even prevent diabetes. It helps to treat high blood sugar and stimulate insulin in the pancreas by healing damaged cells and the blood vessels in and around the pancreas.

It may also treat high blood pressure, kidney and eye disease caused by diabetes and improve vision. Mango leaf tea may also potentially prevent cancers, heart disease, and mental diseases (Parkinson's and Alzheimer's), treat tumors, boost the immune system, and improve digestive. health. More health benefits include treating kidney and gall stones, respiratory problems, stomach ulcers, anxiety, stress, promoting collagen production, and reducing aging signs.

To make mango leaf tea, bring one cup of filtered water to a boil, add a slice of ginger, a dash of nutmeg, and a dash of cinnamon, and boil for five minutes, then add 2-3 clean mango leaves cut into small pieces, remove from heat, cover, and let steep for 5 minutes. Strain, drink, and enjoy. Drinking mango tea on an empty stomach for full results is best.

Guava Leaf Benefits

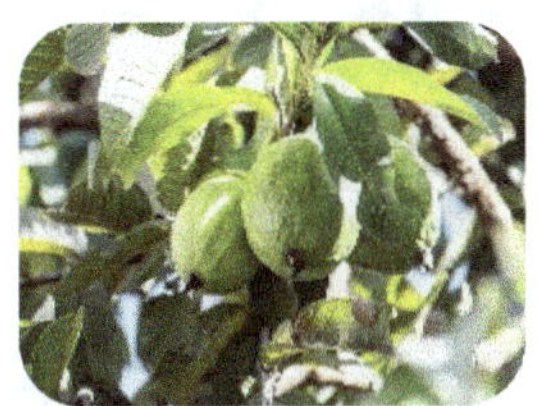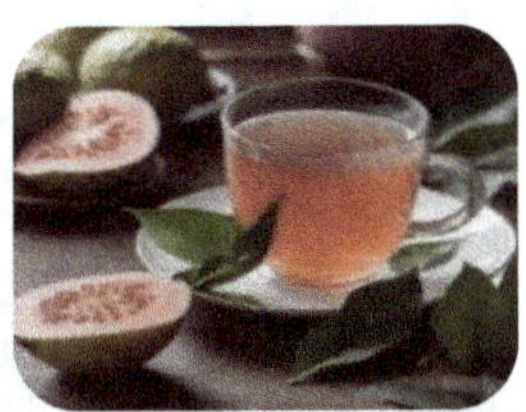

Guava Leaf & Tea (Designed by Pixabay & Freepik)

Guava contains a powerhouse of antioxidants, fibers, nutrients, vitamins, anti-inflammatory, antiviral, antimicrobial, and anti-bacterial properties. Studies have shown that consuming guava leaf tea helps manage blood sugar levels by preventing sugar spikes, improving insulin secretions, and treating other diabetes symptoms. Guava leaf tea can also regulate blood pressure, triglyceride, and cholesterol levels in people prone to heart and cardiovascular diseases.

More good news for people with diabetes is improved blood circulation, reduced risks of eye and brain disease, a healthier immune system, regulated metabolism and prevention of infections and bacterial strains. It also promotes weight loss, stimulates cognitive functions, prevents cancers, and provides relaxed nerves and restful sleep.

To make guava tea, boil one and a half cups of pure filtered water for 2 minutes; add ten fresh guava leaves that have been thoroughly washed, one-half stick cinnamon (a small slice of ginger if you choose). Let boil for 5 minutes, strain, and add flavoring, such as (a slice of lemon, rose water or cinnamon) and sweetener of like stevia or monk fruit extract. Enjoy!

Bitterwood Leaf Tea

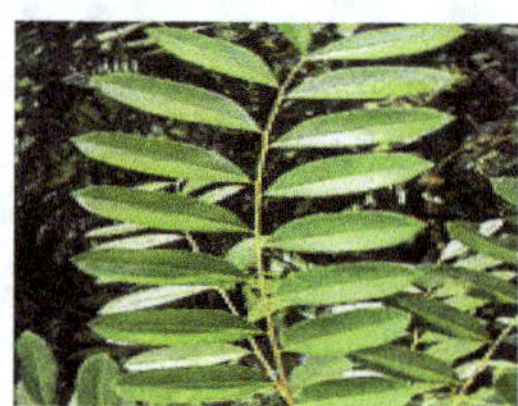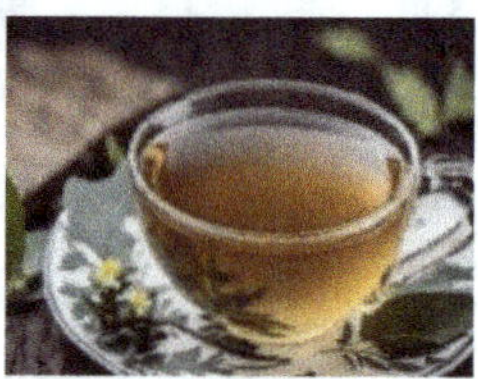

Bitterwood Leaf & Tea (Designed by Freepik)

Bitterwood leaves contain plant compounds that hold a host of impressive health advantages. It is packed with vitamins and minerals and anti-diabetic properties making a plus for people with diabetes. Consuming bitterwood leaf tea may help to efficiently break down the transport of sugar from carbohydrates in the body which is then effectively converted into energy for the body.

This process helps generate and produce insulin which protects the cells and life of the pancreas. More amazing benefits for those with diabetes include cleansing and purifying of the bloodstream, reduced bad cholesterol levels, improved blood vessels and heart health. Seek medical advice about bitterwood leaf tea before consuming it.

Java Plum Leaf Tea

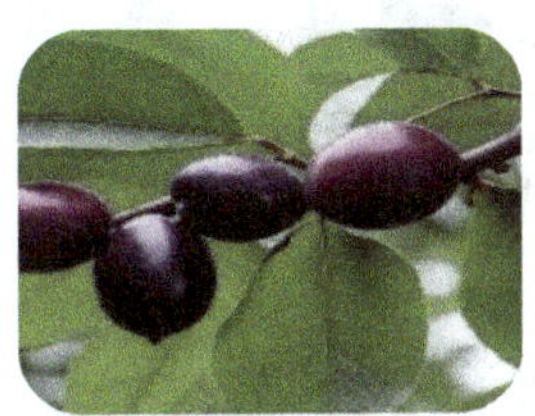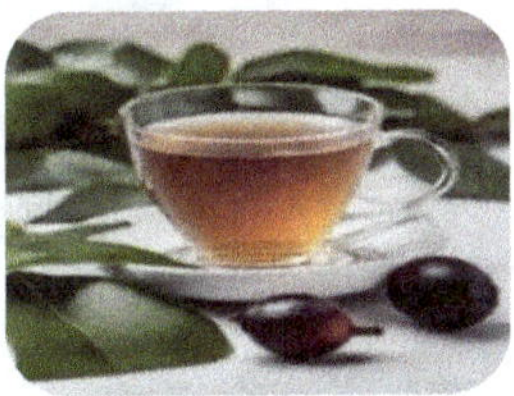

Java Plum Leaf Tea (Designed by Freepik)

Java plum leaf tea is good for diabetes, both Type 1 and 2. It contains compounds, nutrients, antioxidants, anti-microbial, anti-inflammatory, and antibacterial properties. Consuming this tea helps control blood sugar levels because it is effectively broken down into energy in the body and not stored in the bloodstream. Another great benefit for people living with diabetes is that java plum leaf tea may stimulate, produce, and help with the release and response of insulin.

It is said to improve brain, heart, and cardiovascular health and kidney functions, lower blood pressure and cholesterol levels, enhance liver and eye health, protect against cancer tumors, purify the blood, reduce oxidative stress, improve hair health, and promote healthy teeth and gums.

To make java plum leaf tea, wash three java plum leaves and cut them into small pieces. Bring one to one and a half cups of pure filtered water to a rapid boil, add tea leaves, and flavorings such as half of a cinnamon stick if you desire. Boil for 3 - 4 minutes, strain, taste, add sweetener (not sugar) if desired, and enjoy.

Shatter Stone Leaf Tea

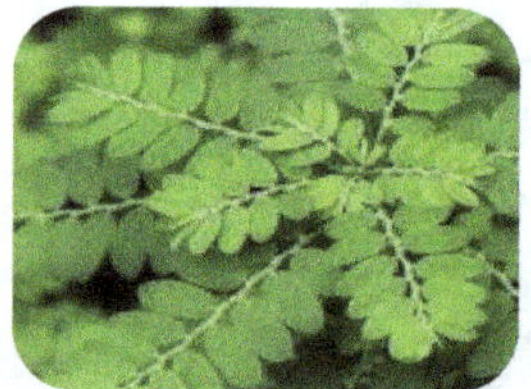

Shatter stone, Stonebreaker Leaves (A Weed in Your Yard)

Shatter Stone, is a yard weed is known by many other names globally: chamber bitter, stonebreaker, gripe weed, etc. It is famous for kidney health anti-diabetic properties. This means that it has the potential to slow the progression of sugar into the bloodstream and thus keep blood glucose levels controlled.

Additional good news for people with diabetes is that it works to keep the heart, eyes, and liver healthy. It contains anti-inflammatory properties which means it helps the body fight against inflammation and protects it from chronic illnesses like diabetes. Its anti-cancer properties protect and prevent cells from cancer and tumors.

Neem Tea Benefits

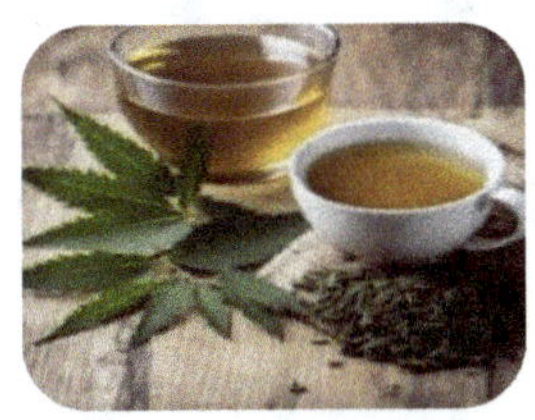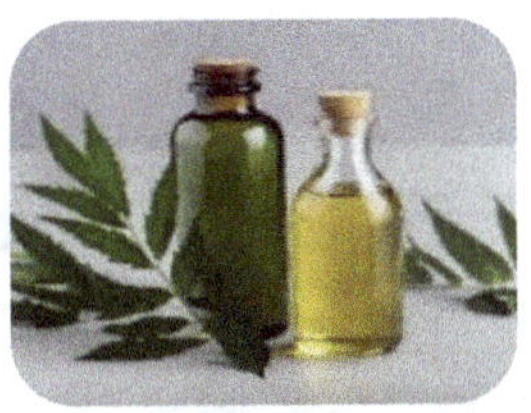

Neem Tea & Oil (Designed by Freepik)

Neem tea is rich in antioxidants, and many plant compounds that when consumed help to lower blood sugar levels and even control diabetes. It may also have the capacity to improve and regulate insulin production and reduce the body's dependency on insulin medications. It also helps lower blood pressure, boosts the immune system, prevents heart disease and stroke, and regulates cholesterol levels.

It effectively cleans the blood, improves blood circulation, enhances eye health, and reduces cancer risks. More benefits are stronger bones, improved digestive health, weight loss, beautiful skin complexion, healthy hair, and oral hygiene; it treats colds and coughs, prevents, or treats the flu, and relieves pain. Neem oil is used for certain skin diseases.

To make neem tea, bring one cup of filtered water to a boil, add two teaspoons of neem leaves, fresh or dried, add a flavoring of your choice such as cinnamon, mint leaf, etc., remove from heat, and let steep for 10-12 minutes, add a slice of lemon and sweetener (I use stevia), strain and sip and enjoy. Warning: Drink in moderation.

African Bitter Leaf Tea

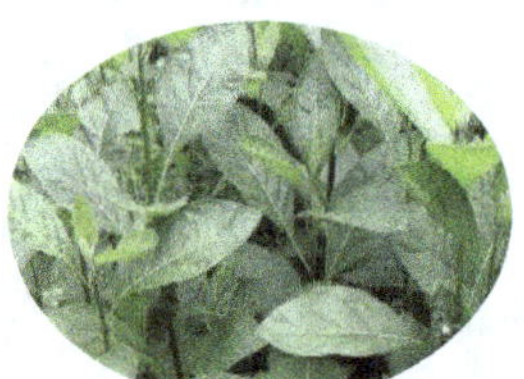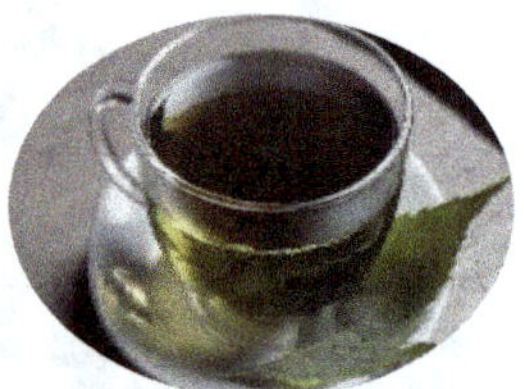

African Bitter Leaves & Tea (Design by Freepik)

Bitter leaf tea is another tea that has health benefits for people with diabetes because of its compounds like phytochemicals, nutrients, vitamins, and other plant properties. It has the potential to reduce blood glucose levels, cleanse the body, especially the liver, and lungs, protect against cancer cells, promote bone and teeth health, and improve metabolism.

Pine Bark/Needles Tea

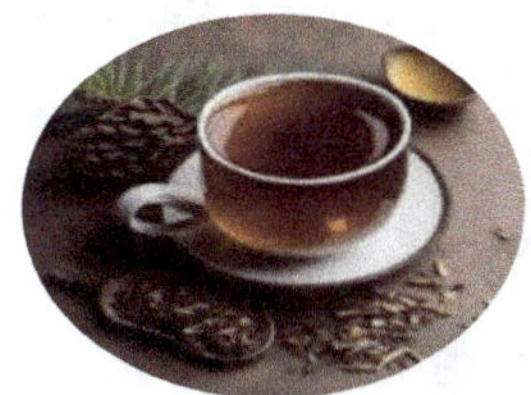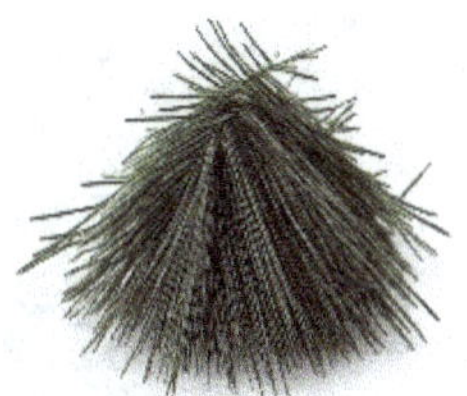

Pine Bark Tea & White Pine Needles (Designed by Freepik)

Pine bark tea extract is packed with health-promoting natural compounds such as phytonutrients, vitamins, and antioxidants (polyphenols) that may have impressive health benefits. Pine bark and pine needle tea are said to have 2-3 times more vitamin C than oranges or lemons. Consuming pine bark/needle tea may regulate blood glucose levels, improve blood circulation, lower high blood pressure, treat metabolic syndrome, and contribute to vision health.

It may also contain anti-diabetic, anti-inflammatory, anti-bacterial, anti-cancer, anti-viral, anti-allergic, and anti-aging properties. It could have the potential to contribute to cognitive improvement, treat Alzheimer's disease, promote cardiovascular health, improve venous flow, boost the immune system, enhance kidney function, and protect against chronic illnesses such as cancers and diabetes.

Although pine bark/needle tea may have these health benefits, it is best to seek professional advice before consuming its tea. White pine bark/needle is the most common of pine bark teas. To make pine bark tea, you use a handful of bark chunks (the cambium layer) placed in about 4-5 cups of pure filtered water (less or more depending on your taste or strength of tea you desire), and let steep unheated overnight, strain, add flavorings and sweetener of your choice.

For white pine needle tea, use ¼ cup chopped needles to 3-4 cups of pure filtered water (less or more depending on your desired taste), boil for 10-15 minutes, let steep for about 5 minutes, and add flavorings and sweetener (not sugar) of your choice. Enjoy.

Banaba Tea Benefits

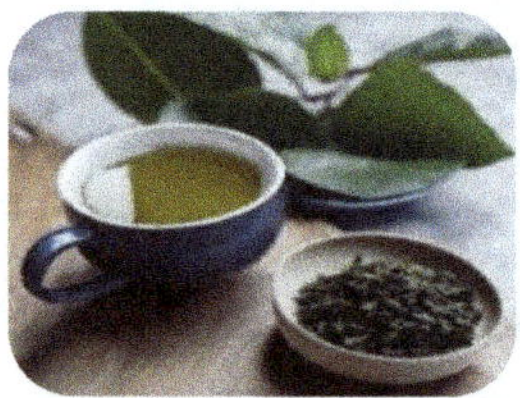

Banaba Tea (Designed by Freepik)

Banaba tea is popular because studies have revealed that it has antidiabetic effects and fights diabetes. Consuming this tea daily may regulate and maintain blood glucose to the normal levels. Banaba's plant substances help to increase insulin sensitivity and transport glucose from the bloodstream to muscle and fat cells for energy.

Banaba is rich in antithrombotic, antioxidant, anti-inflammatory, anti-bacterial, and anti-viral properties. It may also lower cholesterol and high blood pressure, protect the heart and kidneys, prevent lung and liver cancer, and dissolve blood clots. Because of Banaba's plant properties, its tea is used to treat diabetes.

Seek professional advice before drinking Banaba tea. Drink sparingly. To make Banaba tea, bring two cups of pure filtered water to a boil, pour over two teaspoons of fresh or dried Banaba leaves, steep for 3-4 minutes, strain, and add the flavorings and sweetener (not sugar) of your choice.

Gymnema Sylvestre Benefits

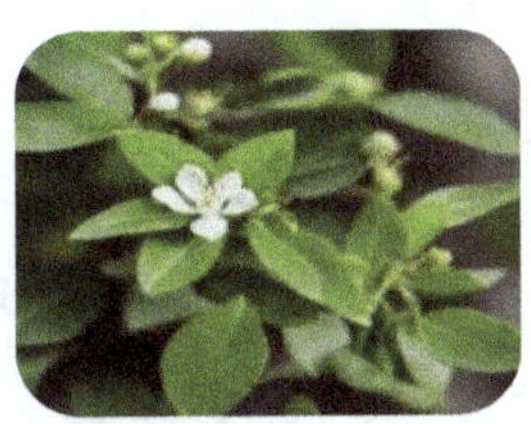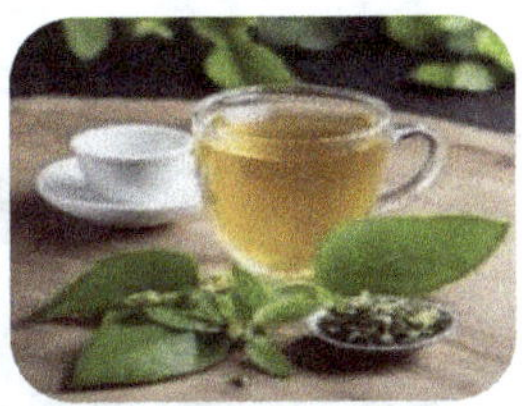

Gymnema Sylvestre Leaves & Tea (Designed by Freepik)

The tea brewed from gymnema sylvestre leaves or "the sugar destroyer" which contain anti-diabetes compounds may have the potential to slowly transport glucose into the bloodstream, which leads to controlled blood sugar levels.

The plant's extract has the potential to stimulate and enhance insulin secretions and promote healthy pancreas cell functions. The conclusion was that blood sugar and HbA1c levels were regulated over time, which could reduce long-term diabetic complications. Use Caution. Drink sparingly; too much can reduce your sugar levels too low. Research and seek professional advice.

To make gymnema sylvestre tea, boil eight ounces of filtered water, add one teaspoon of gymnema sylvestre tea leaves, remove from heat, and let steep for 5-10 minutes. Add flavorings and sweetener (not sugar) of your choice and enjoy.

European Bilberry Tea

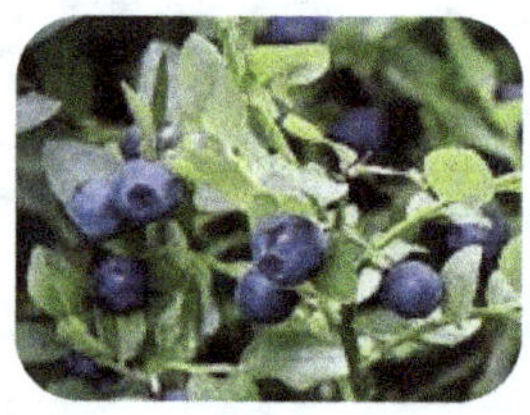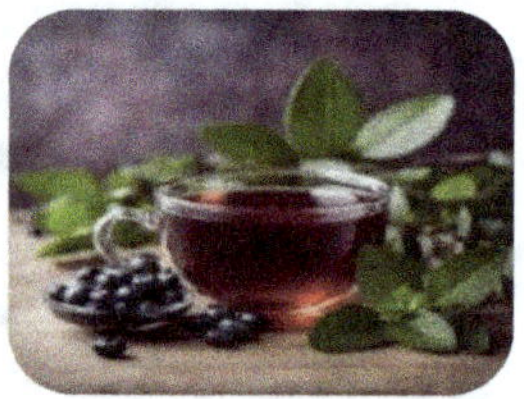

Bilberry Tea (Designed by Freepik)

Bilberry leaves are packed with plant compounds that contribute to overall health. Consuming bilberry leaf tea may help treat and control diabetes and possibly prevent diabetes in those with borderline diabetes. The good news for those living with diabetes is that this tea will slow down the transport of sugar from carbohydrates in the bloodstream and digestive system which leads to lower blood sugar levels. It may also encourage and produce insulin secretions, which lowers blood sugar levels.

Drinking bilberry tea also aids in reducing cholesterol levels, improving blood circulation, promoting cardiovascular and heart health, protecting against eye diseases, preventing liver, and brain diseases, boosting the immune system, and fighting against cell damage due to oxidative stress from free radicals, and reducing the risks of cancer.

Bring eight ounces of pure filtered water to a rapid boil, add one tablespoon of bilberry leaves, and remove from the heat; let steep for 5-8 minutes; strain, add flavorings and sweetener of your choice, and enjoy.

Sorrel/Hibiscus/ Roselle Drink

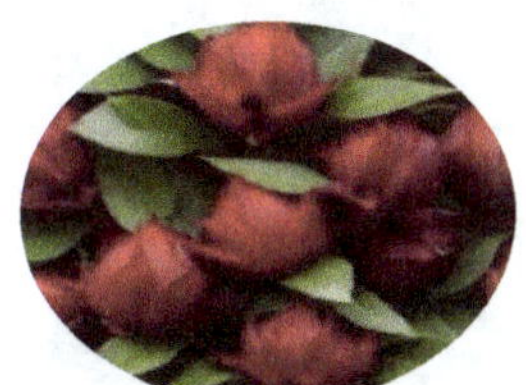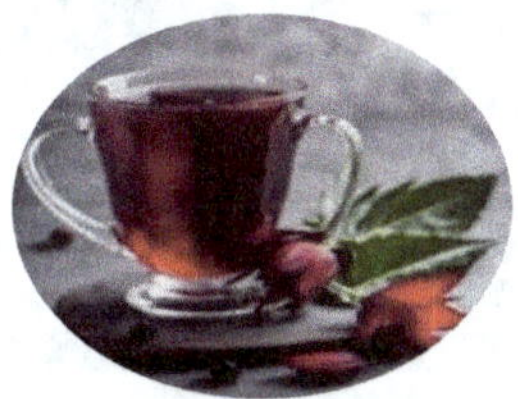

Sorrel/Hibiscus/Roselle Flower & Drink (Designed by Freepik)

Sorrel or hibiscus is packed with powerful antioxidants, anti-inflammatory and anti-microbial properties, it is also loaded with fiber, vitamins, minerals, and nutrients that have super health benefits for people with diabetes. Consuming sorrel drink may have the potential to slowly break down and transport sugar into the bloodstream. This process prevents the spikes in sugar levels and helps to control and manage high glucose and HbA1c levels. In addition, sorrel drink has more health benefits for people with diabetes who are highly prone to other diseases. They can enjoy normal blood circulation, regulated blood pressure and cholesterol levels, protection from all cardiovascular diseases, and prevention of eye diseases associated with diabetes. Furthermore, drinking sorrel regularly reduces the risks of cancers, promotes immune health, improves bone and digestive health, cleanse and purify the body, and boost energy and mood.

Sorrel is a popular Caribbean drink, especially at Christmastime. To brew sorrel drink: Use one cup of dried sorrel, five cups pure filtered water, 1-2 cinnamon sticks, two anise seeds, one two" piece of fresh orange peel, ½ teaspoon grated nutmeg, one teaspoon allspice, four drops of pure vanilla essence, and three whole cardamoms. Boil water, add all ingredients, and simmer for 8 minutes; remove from heat and steep for about 2 hours. Use a sieve with cheesecloth over it to strain the mixture into a tightly sealed jar or pitcher and refrigerate. When ready to drink, pour a glass and sweeten it with stevia, add ice cubes, and enjoy.

Loquat/Japanese Plum Tea Benefits

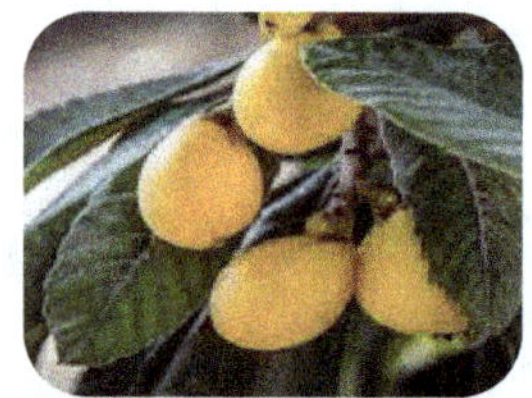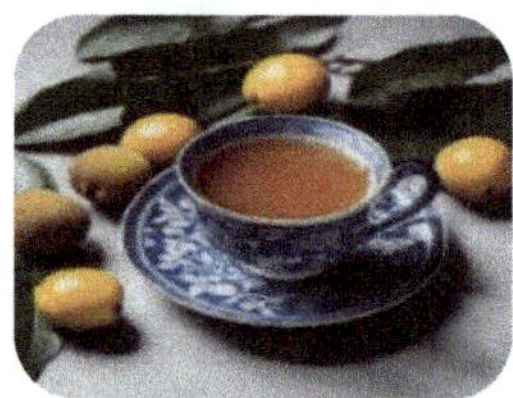

Japanese Plum/Loquat Leaves & Tea (Designed by Freepik)

Research has shown that loquat leaves are a powerhouse of antioxidants, polyphenols, flavonoids, nutrients, and vitamins. It also contains anti-inflammatory, anti-cancer, and anti-diabetes effects. These compounds may potentially prevent and treat Type 1 and Type 2 diabetes by regulating blood lipids and blood sugar levels and increasing insulin levels.

Consuming loquat tea may also protect against cell damage that causes cancerous tumor growth and spread, as well as other chronic illnesses caused by free radicals, reduce the risks of heart and cardiovascular diseases, boost and strengthen the immune system, improve respiratory problems, treat skin ailments, and boost general overall health.

To make loquat tea, you can use both dried and fresh leaves. Add 2 cups of pure filtered water to a pot, wash two fresh leaves around 4 inches long, scrape off all the furry underside of the leaves thoroughly, rewash leaves, remove the middle stem by cutting alongside both sides, rewash leaves, and chop or leave whole (your choice) and place them in the pot. Boil for one minute, reduce heat to simmer for twelve minutes, turn the heat off, cover, and let steep for 10 minutes. Add flavorings and sweeteners (not sugar) according to your taste and choice. **Warning:** Loquat tea is very potent, and one must drink it in moderation. Seek professional advice before consuming loquat tea.

Benefits of Milk Thistle

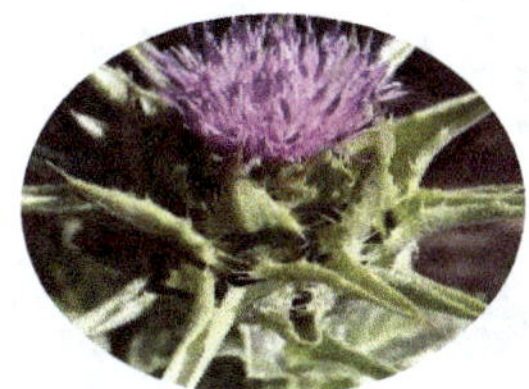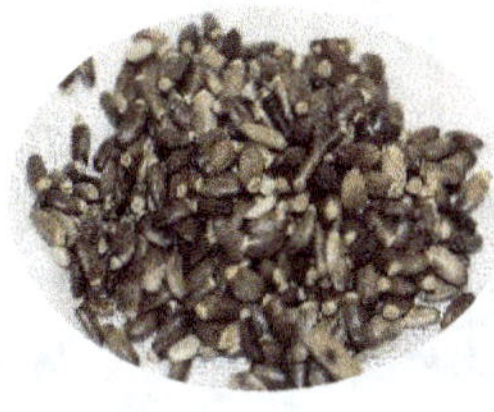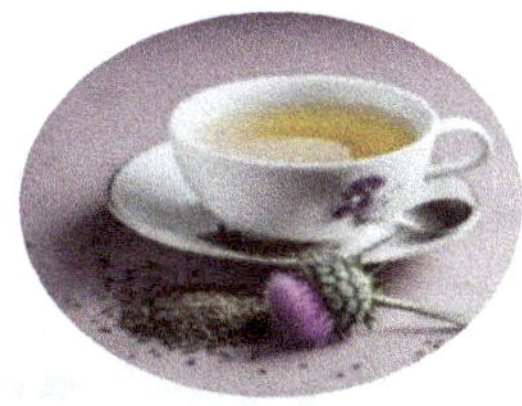

Milk Thistle Plant, Seeds & Tea (Designed by Pixabay & Freepik)

Milk thistle is famous for its ability to treat and protect the gallbladder and liver against diseases. Also called holy thistle, it is rich in antioxidants, anti-inflammatory, and other compounds that may be useful for people with diabetes. Certain compounds in milk thistle can possibly stimulate the pancreas cell to produce insulin which can help lower blood sugar levels.

More possible health benefits for those living with diabetes are reduced cholesterol levels, improved heart and cardiovascular health which is vital because they are at high risk for heart disease. Additionally, the plant's compound may protect against brain diseases, strengthen bone density, prevent cancers caused by oxidative stress from free radicals, and promote weight loss.

For milk thistle tea: measure one cup of pure filtered water to one teaspoon of ground seeds. Boil the water, add milk thistle ground seeds, boil for 30 seconds, remove from heat, cover, and let steep for 8 minutes. Sweeten with stevia and enjoy.

Berberine Tea

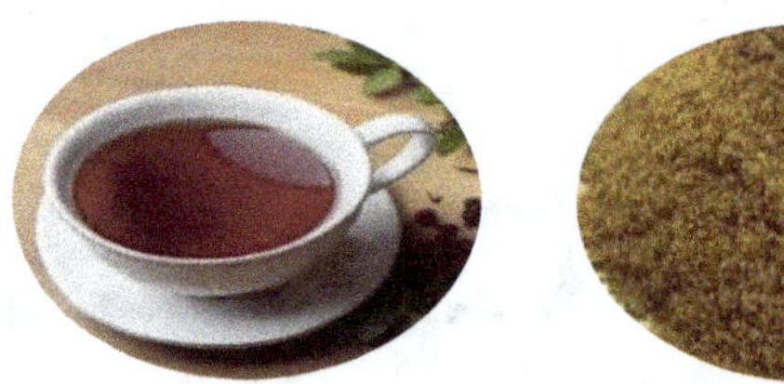

European Barberry Tea and Barberry Root Powder (Design by Freepik)

Research and studies on berberine compounds show that berberine which is found in several plants may be helpful to those living with diabetes. Consuming berberine tea, using the roots of the barberry shrub, may aid the body in increasing insulin sensitivity production, responding positively to insulin, lowering blood glucose levels, promote the healthy breakdown, absorption, and transport of sugar into cells (not the bloodstream) for energy, and regulate metabolism.

Berberine is a plant property that is found in goldenseal, barberry, Oregon grape to name a few. In addition, berberine may contain properties that could reduce sugar production in the liver and even treat liver disease. Furthermore, it supports heart health, widens the arteries, strengthens the heartbeat, and regulates blood pressure, triglyceride, and cholesterol levels.

Research has also shown that berberine tea contains various bioactivities. These include antioxidant, anti-inflammatory, anti-microbial, immune-regulation, anti-aging, and anti-cancer properties. Other health benefits may include the prevention of cancer cells, support weight loss., protection against blood clotting disorders, and enhanced immune functions.

To make berberine tea: use one cup of pure filtered water and one teaspoon of berberine powder. Boil the water, add powder, and stir thoroughly until completely dissolved. You can add flavorings, such as cinnamon, ginger, or lemon. Sweeten with stevia or monk fruit.

Bitter Melon/Gourd Leaf Tea

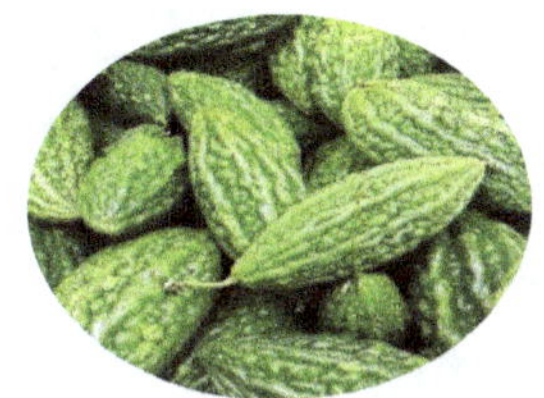 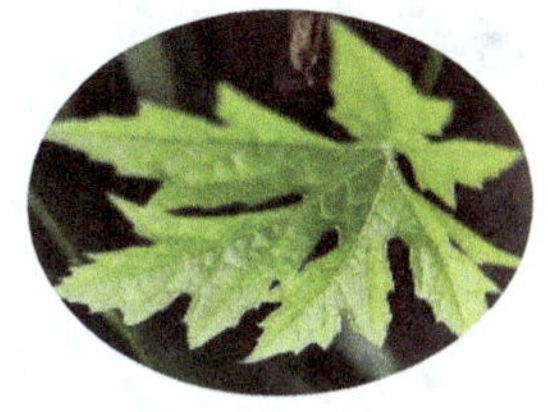 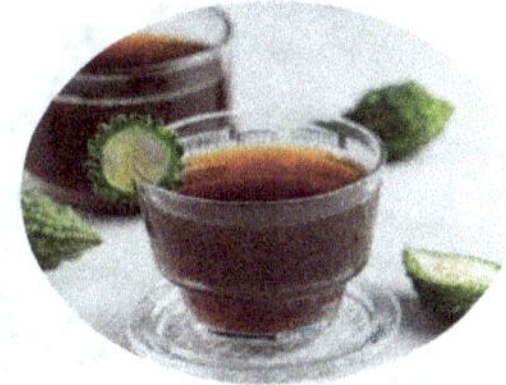

Bitter Melon/Gourd, Leaves, & Tea

Bitter melon or caraille leaves are used to make tea. The plant has a history for its medicinal value and use. It contains polypeptide-p, also known as p-insulin. This is an insulin-like hypoglycemic protein that acts like insulin, which not only helps to regulate blood sugar levels but slows the absorption of glucose into the bloodstream by transporting sugar to the fat cells, muscles, and liver for energy, thus aiding in improved glucose tolerance. Other anti-diabetic properties are charantin and lectin, which also help lower blood glucose levels.

It also contains antioxidants and anti-inflammatory compounds. More health benefits may include blood pressure regulation, removing toxins from the body, treating stomach disorders, and it has antibiotics properties.

For bitter melon tea, use one cup of boiling pure filtered water and one teaspoon of bitter melon leaf, dried or fresh. Cover and let steep for 8-10 minutes; add flavorings such as fresh lemon or lime juice, sweeten with stevia or monk fruit, and enjoy. Before consuming bitter melon tea, ask your healthcare provider if it is safe for you.

Benefits of Stevia

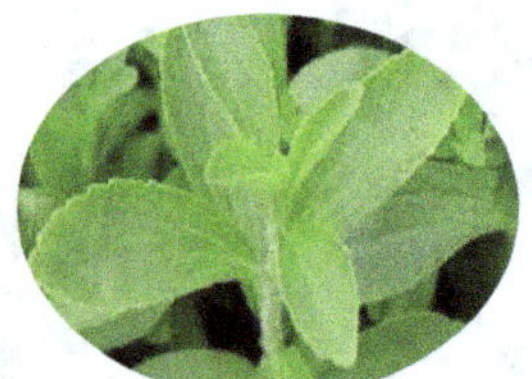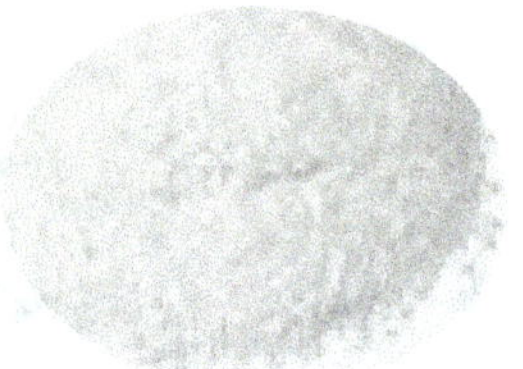

Stevia Leaves & Extract (Free Photos by Vilma)

People living with diabetes should consider using Stevia as a sugar substitute in teas, baking and other foods. It contains several glycosides, phytochemicals, phenolic compounds with potent antioxidant properties, antihyperglycemic, antihypertensive, anti-inflammatory, and therapeutic benefits such as antidiarrheal and diuretic that makes it safe but in purified form and small portions. It has no artificial ingredients and contains antitumor, antifungal, and antimicrobial properties.

Studies of stevia showed that it is free of carbohydrates and its compounds will help to reduce or regulate blood glucose levels, even improve glucose tolerance in the body, and reduce the complications of diabetes. It also has the potential to protect the kidneys, lower blood pressure, improve blood flow to all tissues of the body, promote heart, circulatory, liver, and digestive health, lower triglycerides, lower bad cholesterol and increase good cholesterol, improve blood vessels health, boost the immune system, increase sodium excretion and urine output, reduce the risks of cancers like pancreatic cancer, manage metabolic syndrome, aids in weight loss, allergies, dental health, and protects against oxidative stress.

Additionally, it may be good to include stevia products in children's diets, which may prevent diabetes, obesity, and other health problems. It also protects against acne. Research, ask a professional.

Monk Fruit as a Sugar Substitute

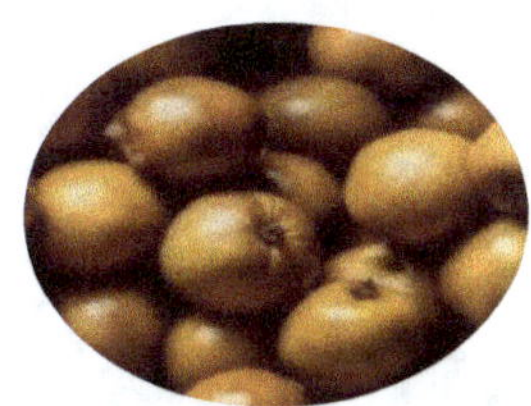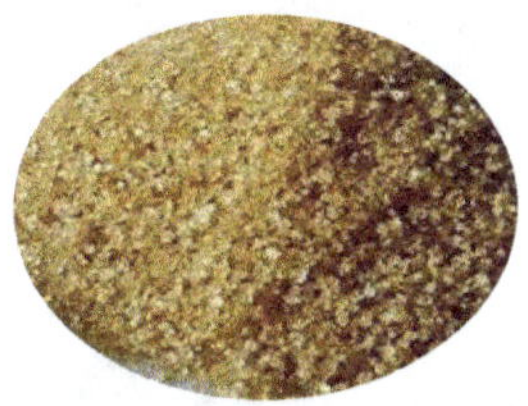

Monk Fruit & Extract (Sugar) (Designed by Freepik)

Monk fruit extract is another natural sugar substitute that those living with diabetes should consider using. This fruit's unique antioxidant properties, called mogrosides, are extremely sweet. However, it will not raise blood glucose levels and has the potential to fight diabetes.

It contains anti-inflammatory and anti-microbial compounds. It may also contribute to heart and cardiovascular health, prevent cancer caused by free radicals, treat high blood pressure, boost the immune system, improve digestive health, protect against kidney disease, fight against infections, and promote weight loss.

Avocado & Extra Virgin Olive Oil

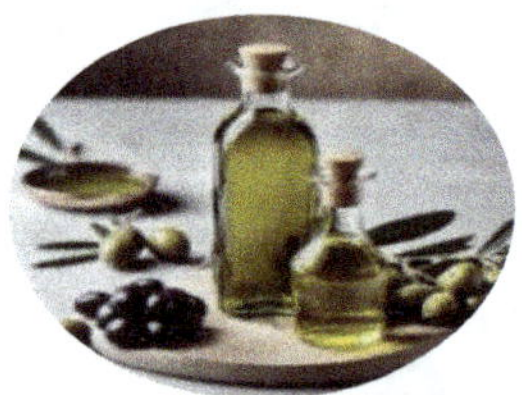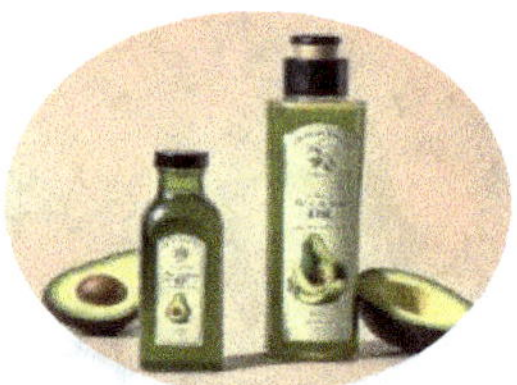

Avocado Oil & Extra Virgin Olive Oil (Designed by Freepik)

Avocado is rich in the healthiest monounsaturated and polyunsaturated fats and has no sugar, so its oil is safe for people with diabetes. Studies have shown that a diet high in monounsaturated and low in carbs may improve insulin sensitivity in people with diabetes. These fats improve heart and cardiovascular health and prevent the risk of strokes.

Another healthy fat oil is extra virgin olive oil which people with diabetes should feel safe to use in daily cooking. The plant's compounds include anti-inflammatory and antioxidants properties that can enhance overall health and protect against diabetic complications. More health benefits include the potential to prevent cholesterol absorption from foods, resulting in healthy cholesterol levels, protection, and prevention of cardiovascular diseases, reduce the risks of brain disease, improve cognitive performance, and protect against blood clots.

Sesame & Rice Bran Oil

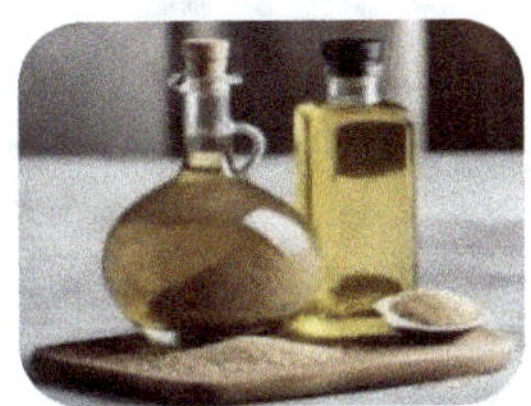 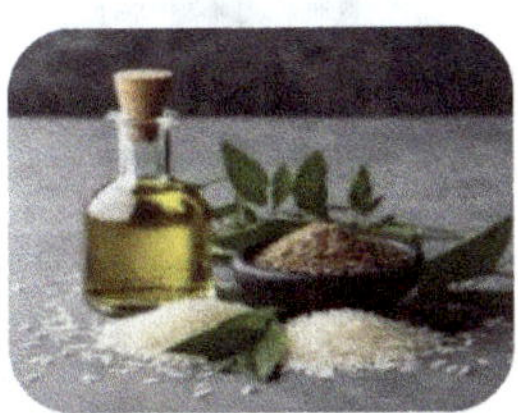

Sesame Oil & Rice Bran Oil (Designed by Freepik)

Sesame oil is loaded with monounsaturated fats and antioxidants which is a smart choice for those with diabetes. Because of its healthy fats and other compounds, it has the potential to help normalize blood sugar and HbA1c levels. Over time, it may help regulate blood sugar to normal levels. It also reduces bad cholesterol and triglyceride levels, which can help prevent heart and cardiovascular disease. It may also prevent plaque from developing in the arteries and strengthen bone density.

Rice bran oil may be another suitable choice for people with diabetes. It proved to lower patients' blood sugar levels and reduced their intake of insulin medication. It also reduces cholesterol and triglyceride levels, thus reducing the risk of heart disease. Using sesame and rice bran oil (mixed) daily for all your cooking, salads, etc., may regulate blood sugar levels to normal levels.

Almond & Walnut Oil

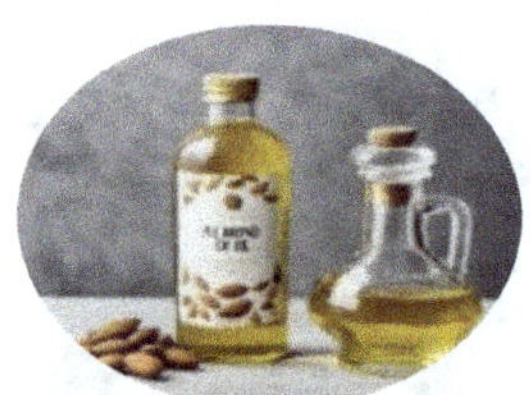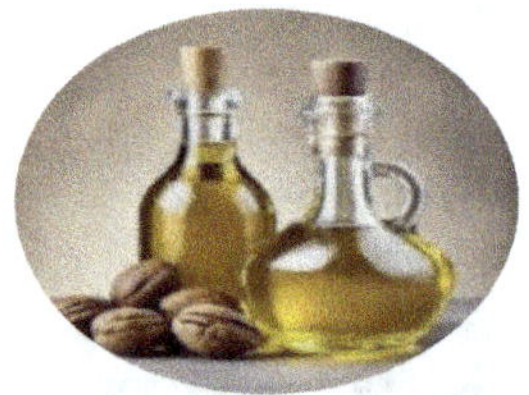

Almond Oil & Walnut Oil (Designed by Freepik)

Almond oil is also a super oil and another excellent choice for people living with diabetes. Its anti-inflammatory, antioxidant properties, and healthy fats help lower blood glucose, blood pressure and cholesterol levels, and lessen the risks of heart and cardiovascular diseases.

Walnuts are rich in healthy fats, and walnut oil is safe for a diabetes diet. Consuming it proved to lower blood sugar and HbA1c levels. It also showed that eating small amounts of walnuts daily can reduce the risk of developing diabetes and prevent diabetes complications.

Grapeseed & Macadamia Oil

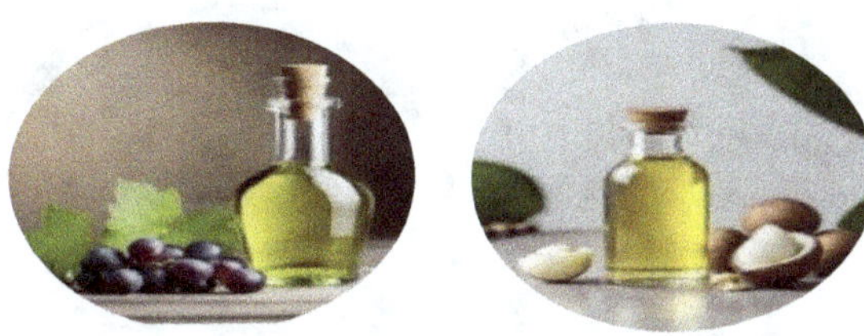

Grapeseed Oil & Macadamia Oil (Designed by Freepik)

Grapeseed is packed with healthy fats and antioxidants, with impressive and amazing health benefits. Intensive studies have revealed that grape seed oil can improve insulin resistance and reduce diabetic complications. It can also improve cardiovascular, heart, eye, liver, and arterial health. It boosts the immune system, improves circulation, prevents cancers, and heals broken vessels and cell membranes. WOW!!!

Macadamia nut oil contains monounsaturated fats and other healthy fats, antioxidants, and nutrients. It is also low in carbs and sugar, which makes it a powerful addition to a diabetic diet. It reduces blood sugar and HbA1c levels and the risk of heart disease, strokes, and metabolic syndrome. Its anti-inflammatory and anti-cancer compounds contribute to health benefits like brain and digestive health and lower the risks of cancer.

Safflower & Peanut Oil

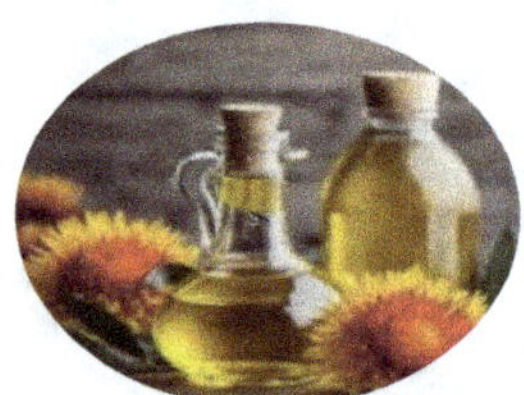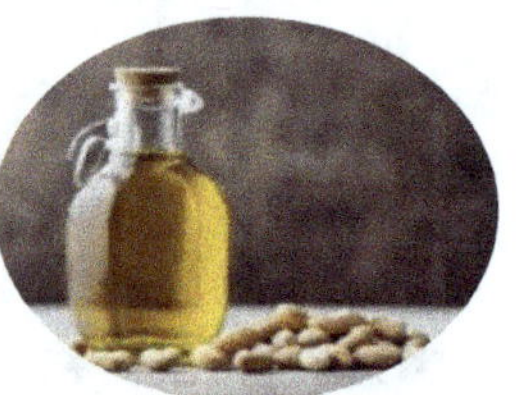

Safflower Oil & Peanut Oil (Designed by Freepik)

Consuming foods cooked with safflower and peanut oil makes them delicious and a healthy choice for people with diabetes. The plant properties and healthy fats offer many health benefits. These include the potential to lower blood glucose levels, prevent heart and brain diseases, regulate blood circulation in the body, control bad cholesterol levels, and enhance immune health.

Hazelnut & Pecan Oil

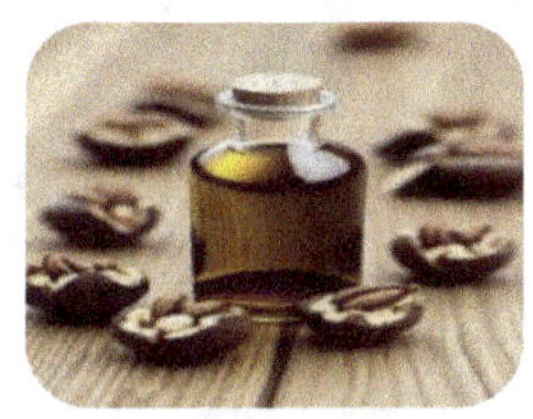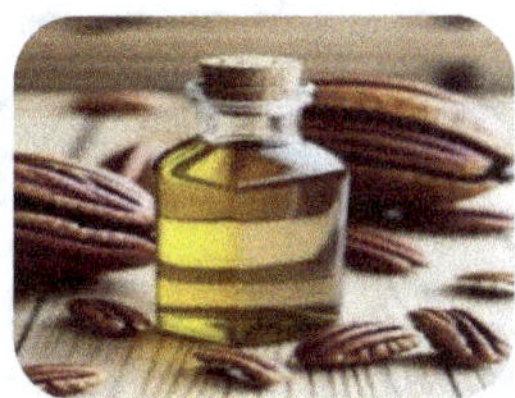

Hazelnut Oil & Pecan Oil (Designed by Freepik)

Hazelnut oil is rich in unsaturated fats, antioxidants, anti-inflammatory, anti-cancer properties and nutrients. Making it a staple in cooking and consuming will promote insulin sensitivity and lower blood sugar, cholesterol, and triglyceride levels, improves arterial health, lowers cardiovascular and heart disease risks, and protect against cell damage that causes cancers.

Pecans are low in glycemic index, carbohydrates, and sugar. It is high in fiber and healthy fats, which prevents sugar spikes by helping slow the absorption of sugar into the bloodstream, which is suitable for blood sugar control. It also lowers cholesterol and blood pressure, markers of a healthy heart.

Chestnut & Coconut Virgin Oil

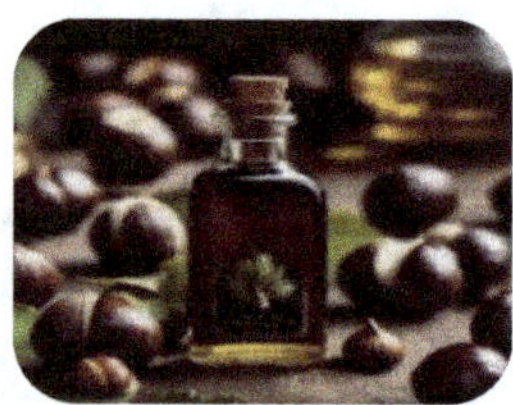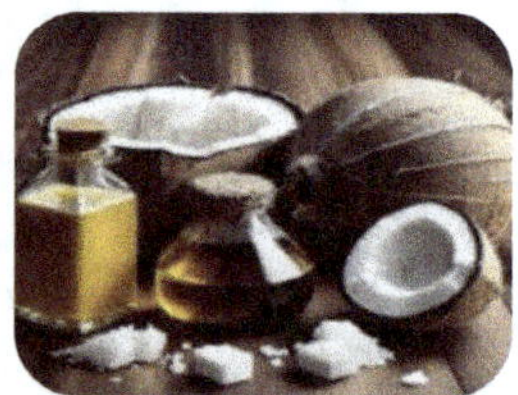

Chestnut Oil & Coconut Oil (Designed by Aitubo)

Chestnuts are rich in antioxidants, anti-inflammatory and anti-cancer properties, nutrients, fiber, and potassium. These compounds in chestnut oil have the potential to protect heart and vision health, lower and manage blood sugar levels, prevent sugar spikes, improve insulin sensitivity and responsiveness to insulin.

Coconut oil is safe for people with diabetes to use. It contains healthy fats, but only if it is raw and unprocessed, such as virgin oil. It can effectively manage how glucose impacts the body. In addition, its fatty acids help sustain insulin performance in tissues and muscles.

Furthermore, it helps keep cholesterol balanced and may decrease the need for insulin therapy in type 2 diabetes. It is effective in glycemic control due to the phenolic compounds and lauric acid, which are rich in anti-inflammatory effects. This is helpful for those diagnosed with diabetes who are prone to develop cardiovascular disease. Coconut oil is great for cooking but must be used according to instructions.

Pistachio Nut Oil, Brazil Nut Oil, Cashew Nut Oil

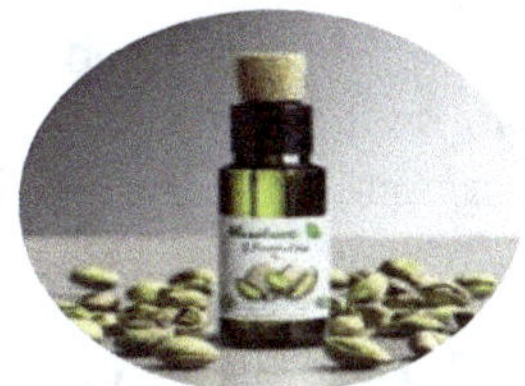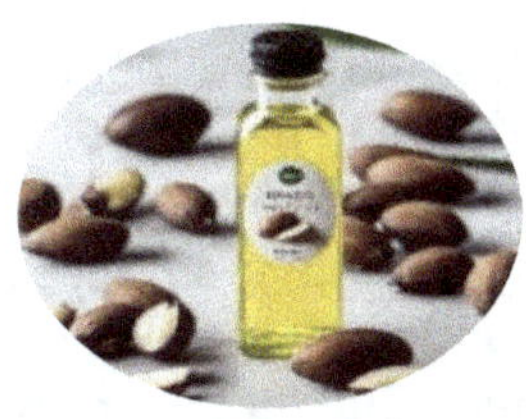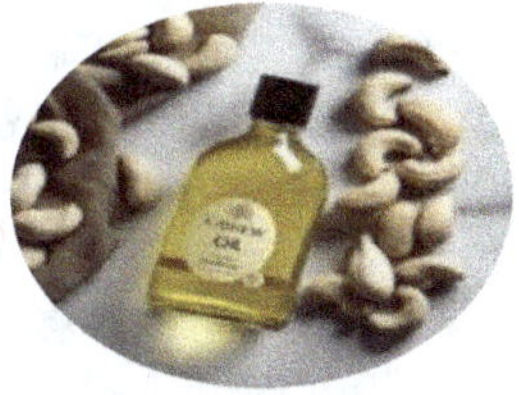

Pistachio Nut Oil, Brazil Nut Oil, Cashew Nut Oil (Designed by Freepik)

Pistachio nut oil is packed with healthy fats, antioxidant and anti-inflammatory compounds, potassium, fiber, and minerals. These compounds help to lower blood glucose, cholesterol, and blood pressure levels in those with diabetes. More good news is reduced risks of cardiovascular diseases, healthy blood vessel functions, and improved digestive health.

Brazil nuts are rich in selenium, monounsaturated fats, antioxidants, magnesium, anti-inflammatory and anti-cancer properties. These properties contribute to improved cholesterol levels and reduced risks of heart disease. Health benefits include improved blood sugar and insulin levels and bone, brain, and immune systems.

Cashew nuts or seeds contain anti-diabetic properties. They offer impressive health benefits, because they are rich in healthy fats and fiber, low carbohydrates, and antioxidant properties. Consuming cashew nuts will help lower blood glucose and insulin levels, improve blood pressure, cholesterol, and triglyceride levels, reduce the risk of coronary disease, and improve brain, kidney, blood, bone, and eye health.

Peppers For Diabetes

Because of their antioxidants and anti-inflammatory properties peppers may have the potential to help with diabetes and improve heart health. Furthermore, hot peppers can lower blood pressure, improve metabolism, and protect cells in the body against cancer caused by oxidative stress from free radicals. In addition, peppers can cleanse the colon, and prevent colon cancer.

Some studies indicate that including hot peppers in your diet can help you live longer. The nutrients in peppers have the power to fight inflammation and obesity. Some names of peppers include jalapeno, banana, chili, habanero, Scotch bonnet, ghost, and Carolina reaper.

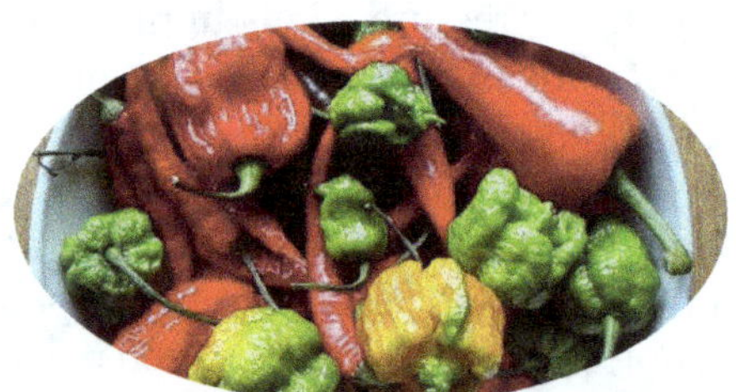

Peppers (Design by Pixabay)

Author's Notes

Free Radicals? What are free radicals?
The antioxidant compounds in the products mentioned in this e-book have healthy components that help prevent cell damage due to free radicals. Free radicals are molecules that cause havoc to tissue and cells, leading to damage and disease. These molecules are unhealthy and are parasitic and love to steal, bond, and multiply, thereby destroying, and damaging tissue and cells in the body.

Where do free radicals come from?
Free radicals come from several factors, such as environmental pollution, radiation, smoking, pesticides, herbicides, certain chemicals, certain foods, and poor health care.

How do we stop or prevent these free radicals?
Antioxidants, antioxidants, antioxidants, and anti-inflammatory properties.

Select foods, fruit, diabetes-friendly drinks rich in antioxidants and anti-inflammatory compounds. This may even reduce the body's aging process.

Glycemic-Index (GI) Foods
Educate yourself about foods best for diabetes; focus on low-glycemic index (GI) foods. Low GI foods release sugar or glucose slowly and steadily into the bloodstream so blood sugar levels do not spike.

Salt Intake
Because people with diabetes are at high risk for heart disease, very low-sodium foods should always be a part of their diet. Another option is no salt or Himalayan salt to barely taste (small amount) when cooking.

There you have it; I blend all the herbs mentioned in this e-book. I am a spice lover, so my food is always spicy. I have experimented with the oils, but now I have a couple of favorites. I have tried all the teas on my journey with diabetes, and I have settled with a few daily. One day, I will drink 3-4 cups of oolong, and the next day, I will try the dandelion and so on. Drinking 3-4 cups of tea each day has helped me manage my diabetes.

Disclaimer

This e-book is for information purposes only. This eBook aims to share information about certain aspects of the products mentioned therein. Every effort has been made to write this e-book as accurately and up to date as possible. There may be typographical errors.

Do not use this book as an ultimate source but as a guide.

The author and the publishers do not profess to be certified experts on the topics mentioned in this e-book. We do not guarantee that the information contained therein is entirely accurate and will not be responsible or liable for any inaccuracies, inconsistencies, or errors.

We shall not have any responsibility or liability to any individual or individuals due to any damage or loss caused or allegedly caused directly or indirectly by this e-book.

Again, this book was written from personal experience by the author and is meant for informational purposes only.

If you choose to use any of the products mentioned therein, please talk to your doctor about it first, especially if you have never used them. Be aware of any allergies before using any of the products.

Author's Letter

Thank you so very much for purchasing this e-book. I hope that you will have great success in controlling your blood sugar and HbA1c levels as I have. It is not an easy task, but I did it and so can you. Eating only foods that are low in carbs, no sugar, very low in sodium, and high in fiber and healthy fats helped me tremendously. But it was a struggle. The teas work miracles. It was difficult for me at first because of the taste of many of them, but I had a mindset, so with a little help from a mint leaf and stevia leaf, and flavorings I made the tea tasty. I have a few favorites. I also have a couple of oil favorites. I do not want to go blind or have a limb amputated or get kidney or heart disease. The foods I used to eat were leading to exactly that. So, I encourage you, for yourself, for those you love, and for those who love you, JUST DO IT. It is worth it, you are worth it, and your loved ones are worth it. I began my mission by taking my medications and eating all anti-diabetic foods, then within six months, my medications decreased, and continued to decrease until about a year later I was medication-free. For those of you who can, I encourage you to grow your herbs and teas. Also buy organic, one hundred% natural, and 100% whole grain or wheat. Avoid supplements, they have been processed and lost their valuable nutrients. To your health and normal blood sugar levels.

Shira

Shira Niru

Author's Profile

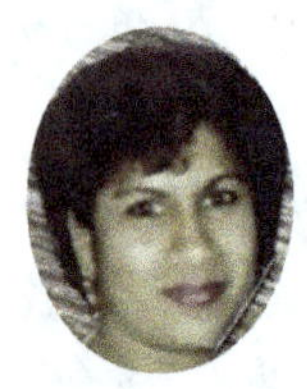

Shira is a retired professional with experience in both the healthcare and business fields. In 1999, she was diagnosed with diabetes. She found it difficult to control her blood glucose and HbA1C levels for years. She began to experience some diabetes complications and made it her life's goal to not allow diabetes to win. She lost her dad when he was 53 years old due to diabetes complications. She knew she had to do something to get her blood sugar levels in check. She returned to and delved deep into her herbal roots (through her grandmother) and educated herself on the nutritional value of foods and drinks that are diabetes friendly. She has been able to control her A1C and blood sugar levels and prevent diabetes complications by eating and drinking the correct foods and beverages.